The Coronin Family of Proteins

Subcellular Biochemistry
Volume 48

SUBCELLULAR BIOCHEMISTRY

SERIES EDITOR
J. ROBIN HARRIS, University of Mainz, Mainz, Germany

ASSISTANT EDITORS
B.B. BISWAS, University of Calcutta, Calcutta, India
P. QUINN, King's College London, London, UK

Recent Volumes in this Series

Volume 36	**Phospholipid Metabolism in Apoptosis**	
	Edited by Peter J. Quinn and Valerian E. Kagan	
Volume 37	**Membrane Dynamics and Domains**	
	Edited by Peter J. Quinn	
Volume 38	**Alzheimer's Disease: Cellular and Molecular Aspects of Amyloid beta**	
	Edited by R. Harris and F. Fahrenholz	
Volume 39	**Biology of Inositols and Phosphoinositides**	
	Edited by A. Lahiri Majumder and B.B. Biswas	
Volume 40	**Reviews and Protocols in DT40 Research**	
	Edited by Jean-Marie Buerstedde and Shunichi Takeda	
Volume 41	**Chromatin and Disease**	
	Edited by Tapas K. Kundu and Dipak Dasgupta	
Volume 42	**Inflammation in the Pathogenesis of Chronic Diseases**	
	Edited by Randall E. Harris	
Volume 43	**Subcellular Proteomics**	
	Edited by Eric Bertrand and Michel Faupel	
Volume 44	**Peroxiredoxin Systems**	
	Edited by Leopold Flohé and J. Robin Harris	
Volume 45	**Calcium Signalling and Disease**	
	Edited by Ernesto Carafoli and Marisa Brini	
Volume 46	**Creatine and Creatine Kinase in Health and Disease**	
	Edited by Gajja S. Salomons and Markus Wyss	
Volume 47	**Molecular Mechanisms of Parasite Invasion**	
	Edited by Barbara A. Burleigh and Dominique Soldati-Favre	
Volume 48	**The Coronin Family of Proteins**	
	Edited by Christoph S. Clemen, Ludwig Eichinger and Vasily Rybakin	

The Coronin Family of Proteins

Subcellular Biochemistry
Volume 48

Edited by

Christoph S. Clemen, MD
Center for Biochemistry, University of Cologne, Cologne, Germany

Ludwig Eichinger, PhD
Center for Biochemistry, University of Cologne, Cologne, Germany

Vasily Rybakin, PhD
The Scripps Research Institute, La Jolla, California, USA

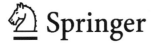

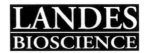

Library of Congress Cataloging-in-Publication Data

The coronin family of proteins / edited by Christoph S. Clemen, Ludwig Eichinger, Vasily Rybakin.
    p. ; cm. -- (Subcellular biochemistry ; v. 48)
  Includes bibliographical references.
  ISBN 978-0-387-09594-3
  1. Microfilament proteins. I. Clemen, Christoph S. II. Eichinger, Ludwig. III. Rybakin, Vasily. IV. Series: Sub-cellular biochemistry ; v. 48.
  [DNLM: 1. Microfilament Proteins. W1 SU14 v.48 2008 / QU 55.3 C822 2008]
  QP552.A27C67 2008
  572'.6--dc22
                         2008020206

ISBN: 978-0-387-09594-3

Published by:

Landes Bioscience, 1002 West Avenue, Austin, Texas 78701, USA
Phone: 512/ 637 6050; FAX: 512/ 637 6079
www.landesbioscience.com

and

Springer Science+Business Media, LLC, 233 Spring Street, New York, New York 10013, USA
www.springer.com

All Rights Reserved
©2008 Landes Bioscience and Springer Science+Business Media, LLC
All rights reserved. This work may not be translated or copied in whole or in part without the written permission of the publisher, except for brief excerpts in connection with reviews or scholarly analysis. Use in connection with any form of information storage and retrieval, electronic adaptation, computer software, or by similar or dissimilar methodology now known or hereafter developed is forbidden.
The use in the publication of trade names, trademarks, service marks and similar terms, whether or not they are subject to proprietary rights.

INTERNATIONAL ADVISORY EDITORIAL BOARD

R. BITTMAN, Queens College, City University of New York, New York, USA
D. DASGUPTA, Saha Institute of Nuclear Physics, Calcutta, India
H. ENGELHARDT, Max-Planck-Institute for Biochemistry, Munich, Germany
L. FLOHE, MOLISA GmbH, Magdeburg, Germany
H. HERRMANN, German Cancer Research Center, Heidelberg, Germany
A. HOLZENBURG, Texas A&M University, Texas, USA
H-P. NASHEUER, National University of Ireland, Galway, Ireland
S. ROTTEM, The Hebrew University, Jerusalem, Israel
M. WYSS, DSM Nutritional Products Ltd., Basel, Switzerland
P. ZWICKL, Max-Planck-Institute for Biochemistry, Munich, Germany

DEDICATION

This book is dedicated to our families and to all scientists in the exciting field of coronin research.

ABOUT THE EDITORS...

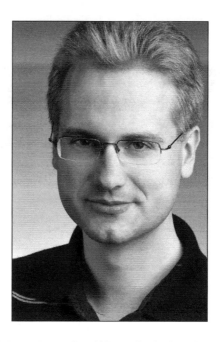

CHRISTOPH S. CLEMEN completed his medical education in 2001 at the University of Cologne, Germany. He received his doctoral degree in Medicine in 2002. In 2003 he obtained his license to practice medicine. Since 2007 he has been a medical specialist in Biochemistry. In 2007 he also obtained his venia legendi in Biochemistry and Molecular Biology at the University of Cologne. He has been a group leader and principal investigator on the Medical Faculty at the Institute for Biochemistry I at the University of Cologne since 2003.

ABOUT THE EDITORS...

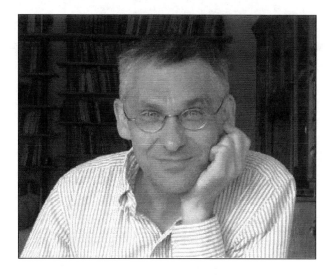

LUDWIG EICHINGER received his degree in Biology in 1989 at Ludwig-Maximilians-University in Munich, Germany. He completed his doctoral degree in Cell Biology in 1992 at the Max-Planck-Institute for Biochemistry in Martinsried, Munich. In 2001 he obtained his venia legendi in Cell Biology at Ludwig-Maximilians-University. He has been a group leader and prinicipal investigator on the Medical Faculty at the Institute for Biochemstry I at the University of Cologne since 1998.

ABOUT THE EDITORS...

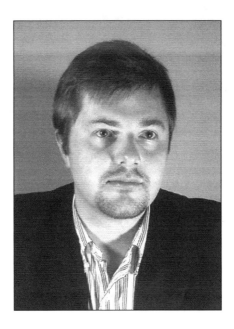

VASILY RYBAKIN graduated with his MSc degree in Immunology from the St. Petersburg State University, Russia, in 2002. He received his PhD in Biophysical Chemistry from the University of Cologne, Germany, in 2005. After a short postdoctoral training at the University of California, San Diego, he joined the Department of Immunology at the Scripps Research Institute, La Jolla, CA, USA as a Research Associate.

TABLE OF CONTENTS

Introduction 1
Christoph S. Clemen, Vasily Rybakin and Ludwig Eichinger

SECTION I: THE WD- AND KELCH-REPEAT SUPERFAMILIES

1. Phylogenetic, Structural and Functional Relationships between WD- and Kelch-Repeat Proteins 6
Andrew M. Hudson and Lynn Cooley

2. Diversity of WD-Repeat Proteins 20
Temple F. Smith

SECTION II: HISTORY, PHYLOGENY AND STRUCTURE

3. A Brief History of the Coronin Family 31
Eugenio L. de Hostos

4. Molecular Phylogeny and Evolution of the Coronin Gene Family 41
Reginald O. Morgan and M. Pilar Fernandez

5. Coronin Structure and Implications 56
Bernadette McArdle and Andreas Hofmann

SECTION III: COMMON AND DIVERSE FUNCTIONS

6. Coronin: The Double-Edged Sword of Actin Dynamics 72
Meghal Gandhi and Bruce L. Goode

7. Invertebrate Coronins 88
Maria C. Shina and Angelika A. Noegel

8. **Evolutionary and Functional Diversity of Coronin Proteins** 98
   Charles-Peter Xavier, Ludwig Eichinger, M. Pilar Fernandez,
   Reginald O. Morgan and Christoph S. Clemen

9. **Role of Mammalian Coronin 7 in the Biosynthetic Pathway** 110
   Vasily Rybakin

SECTION IV: CLINICAL RELEVANCE

10. **Coronin 1 in Innate Immunity** 116
    Jean Pieters

11. **The Role of Mammalian Coronins in Development and Disease** 124
    David W. Roadcap, Christoph S. Clemen and James E. Bear

    Index 137

LIST OF CONTRIBUTORS

James E. Bear
Lineberger Comprehensive Cancer Center and Department of Cell & Developmental Biology, University of North Carolina-Chapel Hill, Chapel Hill, North Carolina, USA

Christoph S. Clemen
Center for Biochemistry, University of Cologne, Cologne, Germany

Lynn Cooley
Department of Genetics, Department of Cell Biology, and Department of Molecular, Cellular and Developmental Biology, Yale University, New Haven, Connecticut, USA

Eugenio L. de Hostos
Molecular Imaging Program, Stanford University School of Medicine, Stanford, California, USA

Ludwig Eichinger
Center for Biochemistry, University of Cologne, Cologne, Germany

M. Pilar Fernandez
Department of Biochemistry and Molecular Biology, University of Oviedo, and Instituto Universitario de Biotecnología de Asturias (IUBA), Oviedo, Spain

Meghal Gandhi
Department of Biology, Rosenstiel Basic Medical Science Research Center, Brandeis University, Waltham, Massachusetts, USA

Bruce L. Goode
Department of Biology, Rosenstiel Basic Medical Science Research Center, Brandeis University, Waltham, Massachusetts, USA

Andreas Hofmann
Eskitis Institute for Cell & Molecular Therapies, Griffith University, Brisbane, Queensland, Australia

Andrew M. Hudson
Department of Genetics, Yale University School of Medicine, New Haven, Connecticut, USA

Bernadette McArdle
Eskitis Institute for Cell & Molecular Therapies, Griffith University, Brisbane, Queensland, Australia

Reginald O. Morgan
Department of Biochemistry and Molecular Biology, University of Oviedo, and Instituto Universitario de Biotecnología de Asturias (IUBA), Oviedo, Spain

Angelika A. Noegel
Center for Biochemistry, University of Cologne, Cologne, Germany

Jean Pieters
Biozentrum, University of Basel, Basel, Switzerland

David W. Roadcap
Lineberger Comprehensive Cancer Center and Department of Cell and Developmental Biology
University of North Carolina-Chapel Hill, Chapel Hill, North Carolina, USA

Vasily Rybakin
The Scripps Research Institute, La Jolla, California, USA

Maria C. Shina
Center for Biochemistry, University of Cologne, Cologne, Germany

Temple F. Smith
BioMolecular Engineering Research Center, College of Engineering, Boston University, Boston, Massachusetts, USA

Charles-Peter Xavier
Center for Biochemistry, University of Cologne, Cologne, Germany

INTRODUCTION

The Coronin Family of Proteins

Christoph S. Clemen,* Vasily Rybakin and Ludwig Eichinger

The coronins, first described in *Dictyostelium discoideum* in 1991, have meanwhile been detected in all eukaryotes except plants. They belong to the superfamily of WD40-repeat proteins and represent a large family of proteins, which are often involved in cytoskeletal functions. Phylogenetic studies clearly distinguish 12 subfamilies of which six exclusively occur in vertebrates. In the present book we have made a sincere attempt to provide a comprehensive overview on all aspects of coronin proteins including history, structure, subcellular localization and function in different organisms. In addition, we also included a general overview on the WD40 family of proteins and the structurally related Kelch family. The book should be of interest for scientists outside the field, but is more importantly intended as a fast and competent guide for newcomers as well as doctoral and postdoctoral scientists to coronin research in all its facets.

The book is divided into four major sections. It provides in the first part an introduction into two superfamilies of proteins with β-propellers, the WD40- and the Kelch-family. Lynn Cooley and Andrew M. Hudson provide evidence that the WD40- and Kelch-repeat families most likely did

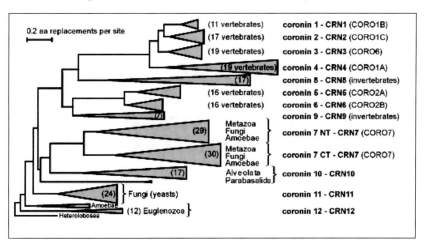

Figure 1. Condensed phylogenetic tree of the coronin protein family. The tree constitutes the basis of a new nomenclature and shows the evolutionary relationship of the twelve coronin subfamilies (CRN1-CRN12). See also chapter II-2 by Reginald O. Morgan and M. Pilar Fernandez.

*Corresponding Author: Christoph S. Clemen, Center for Biochemistry, Medical Faculty, University of Cologne, Joseph-Stelzmann-Str. 52, 50931 Cologne, Germany. Email: christoph.clemen@uni-koeln.de

The Coronin Family of Proteins, edited by Christoph S. Clemen, Ludwig Eichinger and Vasily Rybakin. ©2008 Landes Bioscience and Springer Science+Business Media.

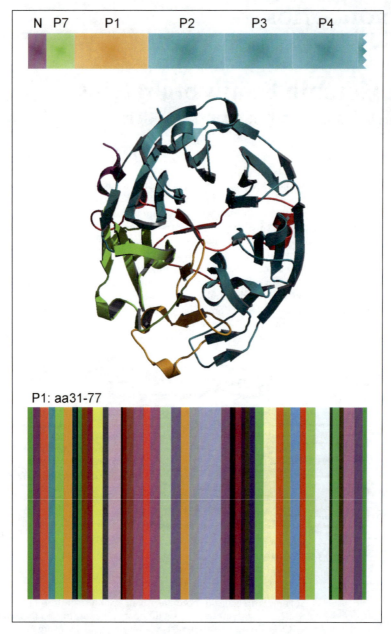

Figure 2. Domain organisation, three-dimensional structure and sequence-into-colour translation of human coronin-1C. Top, True to scale schematic of the domain structure of human coronin-1C; N, N-terminal coronin-specific signature, P1-7, β-propeller blades, C, unique C-terminal region, CC, coiled coil. Middle, top and side view of the structural homology model of human coronin-1C, based on the crystal structure of human coronin-1A. β-propeller blades 1 and 2 that represent an unconventional and a typical β-propeller blade, respectively, are oriented to the bottom (left) and to the front (right). See also Chapter 5 by Bernadette McArdle and Andreas Hofmann. Figure 2 legend continued on the next page.

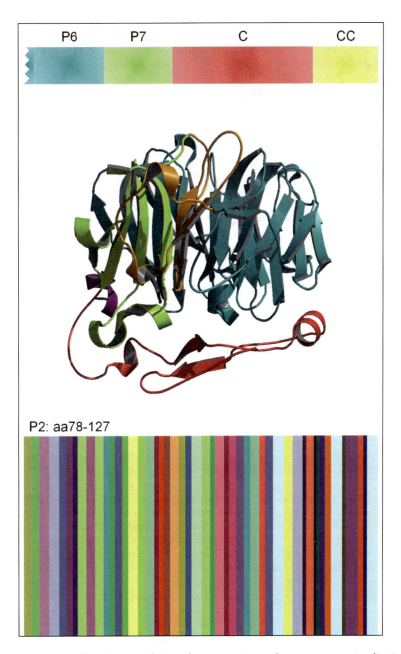

Figure 2, continued. artistic translation of sequence into colour, sequence visualization according to the "iGene-Visions PerZan" colour system (http://www.perzan.de). Each codon is translated into a defined RGB-value. To increase visual harmony in the two images, the width of each bar is coupled to the lightness of its color, the lighter the color, the wider the bar.

not evolve from a common ancestor, although they exhibit similarities not only in their structure, but also in the diverse types of molecular functions they perform (Chapter 1). Temple F. Smith presents an overview on the extraordinary variety of WD40-repeat domain proteins that fold into a β-propeller. This unusual structure provides a platform for the formation of protein-protein complexes that are involved in nearly all the major pathways and organelles unique to eukaryotic cells (Chapter 2).

The second part is made up of three chapters that describe coronin history, phylogeny and its structure. In the first chapter Eugenio L. de Hostos shares with newcomers and experts in the field his personal recollections from the earliest days of coronin research and also provides an overview of the still-developing story of this fascinating family of proteins (Chapter 3). Phylogenetic analysis by Reginald O. Morgan and M. Pilar Fernandez shows that the coronin gene family comprises seven vertebrate paralogs and at least five so far unclassified subfamilies in nonvertebrate metazoa, fungi and protozoa, but no representatives in plants or distant protists. The delineation of 12 subfamily clades in distinct phyla provides a rational basis for revision of the coronin nomenclature, which is intuitive and clear and in accordance with evolutionary history, structural change and functional adaptation. Consequently, they introduce the new symbolic abbreviations CRN1 through CRN12 to unite and renumerate the coronin subfamilies (Fig. 1) (Chapter 4). Due to the weak conservation coronin sequence analyses indicated a variable number of WD40-repeats ranging from four to seven in a single WD40-domain. Structural information revealed the presence of a seven-bladed β-propeller in coronin-1A and a C-terminal coiled coil domain involved in oligomerization. Advanced sequence analyses point to the existence of either seven or 14 WD40-motifs in all coronins. The chapter by Bernadette McArdle and Andreas Hofmann provides a detailed structural description of coronin-1A and presents structural homology models of coronins-1C and -7 (Chapter 5). Figure 2 (top) displays the domain structure of a typical coronin (coronin-1C) with five well-conserved WD40-repeats flanked by two unconventional repeats, which usually remain undetected by secondary structure prediction. The structural differences of a conventional and unconventional β-propeller blade can be appreciated in the structural homology model (Fig. 2, middle). These differences are even apparent in an artistic translation of sequence into colour (Fig. 2, bottom; sequence visualization in a colour system: iGene-Visions PerZan).

The following four chapters deal with the roles of coronins in cytoskeletal dynamics and vesicular trafficking and provide some insight into the development of their function during evolution. The mechanisms by which coronin contributes to cytoskeletal dynamics has remained elusive for many years. Meghal Gandhi and Bruce L. Goode propose a unified model that coronin coordinates actin assembly and disassembly through dual regulatory effects on the Arp2/3 complex and cofilin and spatial targeting of these activities within actin networks (Chapter 6). The chapter by Maria C. Shina and Angelika A. Noegel focuses on nonvertebrate coronins, in particular from *Drosophila melanogaster*, *Caenorhabditis elegans* and the social amoeba *D. discoideum*. Coronin was initially identified in *D. discoideum* and turned out to be an important regulator of the actin cytoskeleton from amoeba to human (Chapter 7). The chapter by Charles-Peter Xavier et al discusses phylogenetic, structural and functional data of the phylogenetically oldest coronin proteins. They describe ancient coronins of unicellular pathogens, chimeric coronin proteins like villidin and in addition they refer to largely unexplored short vertebrate coronins as well as to specific aspects of coronin function not covered in the other chapters (Chapter 8). Mammalian coronin-7, an unusual coronin for which so far no actin binding activity could be shown, was found to bind to the outer side of Golgi complex membranes. It physically interacts with both AP-1 and the tyrosine kinase Src and is recruited to the Golgi upon phosphorylation by Src. This chapter by Vasily Rybakin provides evidence for coronin-7 to act as mediator of cargo vesicle formation in the later stages of cargo sorting and export from the Golgi complex (Chapter 9).

The fourth section is dedicated to coronins in immunity and cancer. The chapter by Jean Pieters describes the current knowledge on mammalian coronin-1A that is exclusively expressed in leukocytes. Recent work based on biochemical, molecular biological and genetic analyses suggest that coronin-1A is involved in the regulation of leukocyte specific signalling events (Chapter 10).

David W. Roadcap, Christoph S. Clemen and James E. Bear present the involvement of coronins in multiple diseases. They highlight possible functions of coronins-1B and -1C in clinically relevant processes such as brain development and neural regeneration. Moreover, coronin-1C is up-regulated in multiple types of clinically aggressive cancer, particularly in the progression of melanoma and glioma (Chapter 11).

In summary, the individual contributions from leading scientists in their respective research fields delineate the established functions of coronins and also highlight active areas of coronin research. Coronins, versatile hubs for protein-protein interaction, play fundamental roles in a variety of significant cellular processes. In recent years it turned out that mis-regulation of coronin expression apparently causes developmental problems and is associated with multiple diseases. Clearly, there is still a lot to be learned about this structurally and functionally fascinating family of proteins.

Chapter 1

Phylogenetic, Structural and Functional Relationships between WD- and Kelch-Repeat Proteins

Andrew M. Hudson and Lynn Cooley*

Abstract

The β-propeller domain is a widespread protein organizational motif. Typically, β-propeller proteins are encoded by repeated sequences where each repeat unit corresponds to a twisted β-sheet structural motif; these β-sheets are arranged in a circle around a central axis to generate the β-propeller structure. Two superfamilies of β-propeller proteins, the WD-repeat and Kelch-repeat families, exhibit similarities not only in structure, but, remarkably, also in the types of molecular functions they perform. While it is unlikely that WD and Kelch repeats evolved from a common ancestor, their evolution into diverse families of similar function may reflect the evolutionary advantages of the stable core β-propeller fold. In this chapter, we examine the relationships between these two widespread protein families, emphasizing recently published work relating to the structure and function of both Kelch and WD-repeat proteins.

Introduction

Experimental approaches aimed at understanding the function of uncharacterized proteins are often challenging. An understanding of known protein domains can provide insights into the possible functions of novel proteins. It has been suggested that WD-repeat proteins might often function as coordinators of macromolecular protein complexes, based in part on the finding that the initial WD-repeat proteins characterized were part of large complexes involved in signaling, transcription, or vesicle traffic.[1] The Kelch-repeat containing proteins initially appeared to mediate interactions with the cytoskeleton since the first Kelch-repeat proteins characterized bind F-actin.[2,3] However, extensive research on proteins with either WD-repeat or Kelch-repeat domains has demonstrated that they perform a very diverse array of molecular functions. Nonetheless, similarities in the structure of these repeat domains and the modular contexts of the β-propellers in both the WD- and Kelch-repeat protein families are useful in predicting the functions of newly discovered members of these families. Several excellent and comprehensive reviews of WD-[4-6] and Kelch-repeat[7,8] proteins have recently been published; here, we focus on recent advances in understanding the structure and function of both families of proteins.

*Corresponding Author: Lynn Cooley—Department of Genetics, Yale University School of Medicine, 333 Cedar St, New Haven, CT 06520, USA. Email: lynn.cooley@yale.edu

The Coronin Family of Proteins, edited by Christoph S. Clemen, Ludwig Eichinger and Vasily Rybakin. ©2008 Landes Bioscience and Springer Science+Business Media.

WD and Kelch Repeats: Sequences, Relationship to Structure and Phylogeny

Kelch and WD repeats consist of repeated sequence motifs with hallmark residues spaced at regular intervals (Fig. 1). In each case, only a handful of residues are consistently conserved (bold residues in Fig. 1 sequence alignments) and even these positions can tolerate substitutions, making the identification of all repeats by sequence scanning algorithms alone difficult. In a number of cases, additional repeats present in a protein were only recognized after structural determination[9] (Table 1).

The structures of WD- (Gβ) and Kelch- (Keap1) repeat domains are presented in Figure 1 (Fig. 1A,B, respectively). While significant diversity has been observed in both WD- and Kelch-repeat sequences, a large number have repeat lengths and repeat spacing similar to those in Gβ and Keap1, making them good representative models. Indeed, even in the structure of Ski8p, a protein containing an unusually long WD repeat, the β-sheet blades can be superimposed on the blades of Gβ with the extra sequence present in loops that project above the surface of the propeller.[9] Overall, both Gβ and Keap1 repeat domains form typical β-propeller folds, with each of the six (Keap1) or seven (Gβ) blades arranged in a circular array around a central axis (Fig. 1 A, B). Each propeller blade consists of four β-strands, which by convention are designated A-D, with the A strand the innermost strand and D the outermost. The twisting of the β-strands gives

Table 1. Structures of WD and Kelch repeat proteins

	Protein	Ref	Species	PDB#	#Repeats/#Blades	Closure Mechanism
WD:						
	Aip1p	27	Budding yeast	1p16	10/14	N-term**
	ARPC1*	36	Cow	1k8k	7/7	N-term
	Bub3p	26,28	Budding yeast	1u4c, 1yfq	4/7	N-term
	β-TrCP*	65	Human	1p22	7/7	N-term
	Cdc4p*	29	Budding yeast	1nex	8/8	N-term
	Coronin 1A	66	Mouse	2aq5	5/7	N-term
	Gβ*	11,12,15	Cow, Rat	1g0t, 1gp2	7/7	N-term
	Groucho1*	67	Human	1gxr	5/7	N-term
	LIS1*	35	Mouse	1vyh	7/7	N-term
	Sif2p	68	Budding yeast	1r5m	8/8	N-term
	Ski8p	9,69	Budding yeast	1s4u, 1sq9	5/7	N-term
	Tup1p	70	Budding yeast	1erj	6/7	N-term
Kelch:						
	galactose oxidase	10	Fungal (D. dendroides)	1gof	7/7	N-term
	Keap1*	13	Human	1x 2j	6/6	C-term
	Keap1*	14	Mouse	1u6d	6/6	C-term

*The structure of the protein has been determined as part of a protein complex or with a peptide ligand bound. #Repeats/#Blades indicates the number of sequence repeats identified by sequence analysis, followed by the number of blades (and therefore, additional poorly-conserved sequence repeats) identified after structural determination. See text for information on closure mechanisms. **Aip1p is organized into two 7-bladed propellers; the N-terminal strand closes the C-terminal propeller and then proceeds to blade 1 of the first propeller. There is no similar closure of the first propeller.[27]

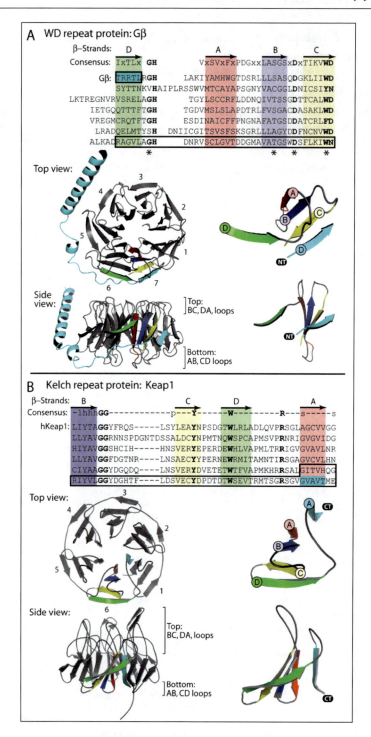

Figure 1. Please see next page for figure legend.

Figure 1, opposite page. Sequences and structures of representative WD-repeat and Kelch-repeat proteins. A) Sequence and structure of Gβ (PBD 1GOT). The sequence begins with the first β-strand of the propeller, excluding the N-terminal extension shown in cyan in the structural models. The top row of the sequence alignment is the WD consensus, though extensive substitutions are common, even among the more highly conserved (bold) residues.[5] Residues marked with an asterisk (*) form hydrogen bonds. In the structural models, the blades are numbered consecutively from N-terminal to C-terminal and the β-strands making up a blade model are lettered A-D from interior to exterior. The boxed sequence in the alignment corresponds to the colored portions of the structures, indicating the location of β-strands A-D of the seventh blade, as wells as strand D of blade 6. Gβ uses an N-terminal strand closure mechanism, by which the N-terminal β-strand (cyan) forms the outer-most strand of the final (seventh) blade, thus closing the propeller. The N-terminal sequence of the repeat continues on to strand A of blade 1. The sequences between the β-strands form loops at the top and bottom of the propeller; these loops are indicated with brackets in A and B. B) Sequence and structure of the Kelch repeats of human Keap1 (PBD 1U6D). The Kelch repeat sequence is largely defined by the conserved GG, Y, W and R residues (bold), though other amino acids are common as well: l = large; h = hydrophobic; s = small; p = polar.[7,8] The boxed sequence in the Keap1 alignment again corresponds to the colored β-strands on the structural models and illustrates the C-terminal closure mechanism, where the C-terminal β-strand (cyan) forms the A strand of blade 1. Since the start and end of repeating sequence motifs are arbitrary, we define the beginning of the repeats as the first residue of β-strand sequence that contributes to the β-propeller domain, making it easier to see how the sequence repeats contribute to structure. For the WD repeat, this is the same definition that is commonly used.[1,5] However, note that the Kelch repeat sequence is sometimes defined as beginning at the "A" β-strand. Sequence repeats were aligned manually and structural views were prepared using MacPyMOL.[63]

the propeller a tapered toroidal appearance. By convention the "top" of the structure is defined as the narrower surface (Fig. 1).

WD sequence repeats are approximately 40 amino acids in length and the most conserved residues are a Gly-His (GH) dipeptide near the beginning of each repeat, as well as the eponymous Trp-Asp (WD) dipeptide that terminates the repeat.[5] The first structure determination of a WD-repeat protein was that of Gβ, the beta subunit of a heterotrimeric G-protein complex[10-12] and this structure revealed the relationship of the repeat sequence to the β-propeller structure. The β-strands are offset relative to the blade structure of the propeller so that the first β-strand of the sequence repeat is the outermost strand of one blade, while the next three β-strands in the sequence make up the three inner β-strands of the next blade. This is illustrated in Figure 1, where the β-strands of the final sequence repeat (boxed sequence) are displayed in color on the structural model. The RAGVL sequence makes up the outer strand (strand D) of repeat 6, while strands A-C comprise the three inner strands of repeat 7. This offset arrangement of β-strands provides a mechanism to stably close the barrel structure; the seventh and final blade of the propeller is comprised of the three C-terminal β-strands, while the outermost β-strand is the N-terminal sequence at the beginning of the seven repeats. This closure mechanism has been termed N-terminal strand closure and is illustrated in Figure 1A, where the N-terminal β-strand sequence TRRTL is highlighted in Cyan in the sequence and on the structural models. N-terminal strand closure has been observed for all WD-repeat structures determined to date (Table 1).

Kelch repeats were first identified in the *Drosophila* cytoskeletal regulatory protein Kelch.[3] They possess a consensus sequence distinct from that of WD-repeats and, at 44-56 amino acids in length, are generally slightly longer (Fig. 1B). Signature residues include a diglycine doublet near the beginning, followed by reasonably well-conserved Tyr, Trp and Arg residues at regular spacing throughout the remainder of the repeat. The structures of fungal galactose oxidase[10] and the human[13] and murine[14] Keap1 Kelch-repeat domains have been determined. The overall structural organization of the Keap1 Kelch repeats is quite similar to that of Gβ and other β-propellers. Like Gβ, the sequence repeat is offset relative to the structural repeat and this again provides a mechanism for structurally closing the barrel. However, instead of the N-terminal strand closure mechanism used by WD repeat proteins, Keap1 uses C-terminal strand closure, where the C-terminal β-strand forms the interior-most strand of the first propeller blade (cyan in the sequence alignment and structures in Fig. 1B). In contrast, galactose oxidase uses N-terminal strand closure,[10] demonstrating that either mechanism is possible for Kelch repeat proteins. However, sequence analysis revealed that three quarters of the human Kelch-repeat proteins are predicted to use C-terminal strand closure.[8]

For both WD- and Kelch-repeat proteins, the more highly conserved residues that define the repeat sequences are important for the structural integrity of the β-propeller. In WD-repeat proteins, a conserved tetrad of amino acids (Fig. 1A, asterisks) is hydrogen bonded.[12,15] In the Kelch structures, the highly conserved diglycine doublet occurs after the B strand where the backbone adopts conformation that strongly favor glycines.[16] The conserved Tyr, Trp and Arg residues in the C-terminal portion of the repeat all participate in hydrogen bonding interactions important for structural stability. The signature residues of WD and Kelch repeats thus are important for structural integrity, while the more variable sequences present in the loops create diverse surfaces that likely determine the functional characteristics of individual WD- and Kelch-repeat proteins.

Despite the remarkable structural similarity, WD-repeat and Kelch-repeat proteins are unlikely to have evolved from a single common ancestor, but instead appear to have evolved along parallel paths.[17,18] β-propeller domain proteins likely arose from a single copy of the sequence repeat encoding a four-stranded β-sheet that underwent duplication events to generate a series of tandem repeats. Subsequently, the individual repeats likely diverged through sequence insertions, deletions and polymorphisms, leaving only the relatively few conserved residues important for maintaining the β-propeller fold.[18-20] Interestingly, the protein tachylectin-2 is a five-bladed β-propeller made up of highly homologous sequence repeats distinct from WD or Kelch repeats. This suggests that tachylectin-2 is a relatively recent descendant from an ancestral sequence repeat.[21] In contrast, the degenerate WD- and Kelch-repeat sequences clearly arose much earlier in evolution.

Both WD- and Kelch-repeat β-propellers are modular in nature. The β-propeller module can be present alone or at the amino- or carboxy-terminus of proteins that contain other structural motifs. The most common accompanying structural motifs mediate dimerization or oligomerization, or association with cullin-based ubiquitin E3 ligases (Table 2). In addition, examples have been found of proteins that contain two (or possibly more) β-propellers connected by linkers. The variety of modular contexts of β-propellers reflects the functional diversity of the proteins that contain them.

Further Insights from Structures of WD- and Kelch-Repeat Proteins

In the past few years the structures of more than 12 WD-repeat proteins have been solved (Table 1), including a number as part of protein complexes or with peptide ligands bound. In addition, the structures of the mammalian Keap1 Kelch-repeat domains represent important additions to the sole previous Kelch-repeat structure, that of the galactose oxidase, which contains seven Kelch repeats. The vast majority of Kelch-repeat proteins in metazoans,[8] as well as those that have been functionally characterized in *Arabidopsis*,[22-24] contain six Kelch repeats and exhibit closer overall homology to Keap1 than to galactose oxidase. Thus the large number of WD-repeat protein structures, together with the few Kelch-repeat domain structures available, allows structural comparisons to be made.

A wide range of repeat numbers has been reported for both WD- and Kelch-repeat proteins. Numbers of WD repeats range from 4 to 14 in characterized proteins and a predicted protein with 18 WD repeats exists in the Pfam database.[25] Recent WD-repeat structures provide important insights about how these proteins fold. First, WD proteins with fewer than seven identified repeats likely have additional "hidden" repeats that bring the number of blades to seven. This was the case for six WD-repeat proteins whose structures have been solved (Table 1) and in most cases, once the structure was determined it was possible to identify highly degenerate WD repeats within the protein sequence.[9,26-28] Second, a number of WD-repeat proteins have been described containing greater than 10 tandem repeats and it was not clear whether these form single large propellers or fold into multiple smaller discrete propeller domains. The structure of Aip1p, an F-actin interacting protein that was reported to contain 10 WD repeats, revealed a "clamshell" shaped structure consisting of two 7-bladed propellers.[27] In this case, the large number of repeats did not indicate a correspondingly large number of blades in a single propeller. These results suggest that there is an inherent stability in, or selection for, seven-bladed WD-repeat β-propellers. However, this is clearly not a rigid requirement: the WD-repeat domain in budding yeast Cdc4p contains eight repeats and forms an 8-bladed propeller.[29] In addition, Sec13p, a COPII vesicle coat protein, contains six WD repeats and has no additional sequence that could harbor additional cryptic repeats and so most likely folds into a 6-bladed propeller.[30]

The number of Kelch repeats that can be identified in a protein also varies, though not to the same extent as WD-repeat proteins. The structures of galactose oxidase and the Kelch-repeat domain of Keap1 have seven and six blades, respectively. The horseshoe crab F-actin crosslinking protein α-scruin has 12 Kelch repeats, but they are in two clusters, each with six tandem repeats at either end of the protein separated by an intervening sequence. Cryo-EM data indicate that α-scruin has a "dumbbell" conformation, apparently with six-bladed β-propellers at either end of the protein.[31] Thus, it appears that Kelch repeats form 6 or 7 bladed β-propellers, with 6 being more common. However, there are some examples of predicted proteins with fewer than six Kelch repeats[8] for which no structural information is available. In addition, a large family of Kelch-repeat proteins has been identified in the *Arabidopsis* genome, where the proteins clearly contain only four repeats.[32,33] These proteins all contain N-terminal F-boxes and thus are predicted to function as substrate-specific adapter proteins in ubiquitin E3 ligases. However, whether the Kelch repeats fold into typical β-propeller proteins is not clear. The predicted *Arabidopsis* F-box/4xKelch-repeat proteins also contain two absolutely conserved cysteine residues, raising the possibility that disulfide bridges may play a role in forming a modified Kelch-repeat propeller-like structure.[32]

Perhaps the most significant differences between the WD- and Kelch-repeat derived β-propellers are the sequences that connect the β-strands. These sequences emerge at the top or bottom of the propeller and therefore determine the characteristics of these surfaces. In many WD-repeat proteins, the loops between β-strands A and B (AB loops; top surface), as well as the BC loops (bottom surface), are short (3-5 amino acids) and show little variability. In contrast, the other two β-strand connecting loops, the CD (bottom) and DA (top) loops, are longer and more variable and create a significant portion of the accessible surface on the top and bottom of the propeller (Fig. 1A).

Table 2. β-propeller domain organization in representative proteins

	WD	Kelch
N-terminal βProp		
CT-oligomeriztion	Coronin	Kel1p, Kel2p, Tea1p
CT-misc.	CAF-1 (p60 subunit)	Rag2, Ral2p, LZTR-1
	HirA proteins	
C-terminal βProp		
NT-Fbox	Cdc4, βTrCP, others	FBox-Kelch proteins
	(≥ 20 predicted in animals)	(≥ 40 predicted in plants)
NT-BTB	-	BTB-Kelch family
		(≥ 40 predicted in humans)
NT-oligomeriztion	LIS1, Tup1p, Groucho/TLE	Muskelin
	CstF-50	
NT-misc	Gβ	Galactose oxidase
βProp alone	ARPC1, Bub3p, Sec13p	p40
Multiple βProps	Aip1p	α-scruin, β-scruin
	Lgl (predicted multiple props)	
βProp within large multi-domain proteins	p532 (aka p619)	HCF-1, HCF-2, Attractin/Mahogany

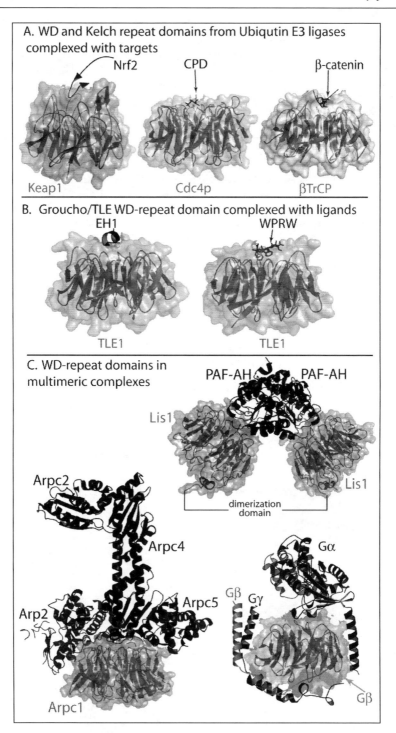

Figure 2. Please see next page for figure legend.

Figure 2, opposite page. Structures of WD- and Kelch-repeat β-propellers cocrystalized with ligands. In all cases, the WD- or Kelch-repeat domain is gray while bound peptides or proteins are shown in black. To facilitate viewing the binding interfaces, the β-propeller proteins are also presented with transparent surface projections. A) β-propellers from ubiquitin E3 ligases complexed with peptides derived from their targets. On the left is the structure of the Keap1 Kelch-repeat domain complexed with a peptide derived from Nrf2. Nrf2 is the only known binding partner of the Keap1 Kelch-repeat domain and is a targeted for ubiquitin-mediated destruction by a Cul3-Keap1 ubiquitin ligase. WD-repeat domains of Cdc4p and βTRCP are shown, also complexed with peptides derived from their biological targets; N-terminal residues were removed for clarity. B) Structures of Groucho1 bound to two different peptides derived from distinct Groucho1 binding partners. C) WD-repeat proteins that have been crystallized as part of a multiprotein complex. LIS1 is shown complexed with a PAF-AH dimer; LIS1 is also a dimer, though its N-terminal dimerization domains were not visible in the crystal structure. ARPC1 is shown with other components of the Arp2/3 complex that make contacts with ARPC1. Arp3 and Arpc3 are not shown and only part of Arp2 is resolved in this structure. Gβ is shown complexed with Gα and Gγ. All structural views were prepared using MacPyMOL[63] and structural coordinates are listed in Table 1, except for the Arp2/3 complex, where PBD 2p9k was used.[64]

For Kelch-repeat proteins, the two loops on the bottom of the propeller (the AB and CD loops) are both short and well conserved. Instead, the longer and more variable loops (the BC and DA loops) both extend from the top surface. Thus the longer loops of the Keap1 propeller present a more elaborate top surface when its side view is compared with that of Gβ (Fig. 1B).

The observation that WD-repeat proteins have variable loops on both the top and bottom surfaces suggests an ability to use both surfaces for protein-protein interaction; indeed, some WD-repeat proteins that have co-evolved in multi-protein complexes do have interactions on both surfaces and even on the sides (see below). However, existing data do not support this idea as a general rule. Several structures have been solved with a WD-repeat protein bound to a known interacting protein in which the protein-protein binding interfaces are exclusively on the top face of the β-propeller (Fig. 2A,B). For example, the WD-repeat domains of Cdc4p and β-TrCP are substrate recruitment domains for ubiquitin E3 ligases and in each case, the bound peptide makes extensive contacts with residues in the variable loops that extend from the top surface. In addition, the WD-repeat domain of the Groucho/TLE transcriptional repressor protein TLE1 has been crystallized with peptides whose sequences are derived from two distinct classes of Groucho/TLE interacting proteins.[34] Both peptides bind on the top surface in the pocket created where the central channel of the propeller opens and both peptides form binding interactions with residues from each of the seven propeller blades. LIS1 has a well-characterized function regulating the microtubule motor dynein and in vertebrates is also known to associate with the dimeric enzyme Platelet-Activating Factor acetylhydrolase (PAF-AH). Murine LIS1 was crystallized in complex with PAF-AH and this structure revealed that the LIS1 WD-repeat domain makes extensive contacts with PAF-AH exclusively through its top face (Fig. 2C).[35] Binding competition studies and mapping of conserved surface-exposed residues suggest that other LIS1 ligands compete with PAF-AH for binding to the top surface of the LIS1 β-propeller.

Two WD-repeat proteins, Gβ and ARPC1, were crystallized as parts of large multiprotein complexes (Fig. 2C).[15,36] ARPC 1 is a component of the F-actin nucleating Arp2/3 complex and Gβ is an integral component of the G-protein heterotrimer. Both of these protein complexes are evolutionarily ancient, being present throughout all eukaryotic phyla. These structures reveal that within these complexes, WD-repeat proteins are indeed multivalent proteins making simultaneous contacts with multiple proteins. The Gα and Gγ proteins make extensive contacts with the sides and top of the Gβ propeller (Fig. 2C). The Arp2/3 components that bind ARPC1 make extensive contacts with top surface of the propeller; only the actin-related protein Arp2 is associated with the side of the propeller (Fig. 2C). However, additional known Arp2/3 interactions likely involve the bottom surface of the β-propeller. These include F-actin and Arp2/3 activating proteins of the Scar/Wasp family (discussed in reference 37). Indeed, there is a large patch of highly conserved surface-exposed residues on the bottom face of the ARPC1 β-propeller that likely forms an interaction surface.[37]

The structures of the Kelch-repeat domains from the mammalian Keap1 proteins were solved with peptides derived from Nrf2 (Fig. 2A).[14,38] Like Cdc4p and β-TrCP, Keap1 is also a substrate-targeting component for a cullin-based ubiquitin E3 ligase and the only known target is the transcription factor Nrf2.[39-41] Like the WD-repeat based E3 ligase substrate adaptors, the Nrf2 peptide is present in a pocket created by the channel on the top surface of the propeller. The Nrf2 peptide makes contacts with residues in the CB and DA loops from all but the third blade.

The structural information currently available suggests that β-propellers can act as a scaffold for multiple protein interactions or form a monovalent interaction surface. In cases where the β-propellers are components of ancient protein complexes such as the Arp2/3 complex or heterotrimeric G-proteins, multiple interactions have evolved. However, other WD- and Kelch-repeat proteins, notably the ubiquitin E3 ligase substrate adaptors, bind only one or several similar sequences. This may explain the expansion of WD- and Kelch-repeat proteins in higher eukaryotes; the β-propellers form a rigid structural domain, perhaps providing a stable platform on which the surface loops can evolve to form distinct protein-protein interaction domains.

Major Functional Classes of WD- and Kelch-Repeat Proteins

Both WD- and Kelch-repeat proteins have been demonstrated to participate in a wide variety of cellular and biochemical functions and new functions for these proteins will certainly be ascribed as additional proteins are functionally characterized. Comprehensive enumerations of functional classes for both WD- and Kelch-repeat proteins have been presented for both classes previously.[1,6,7] However, an examination of the molecular functions of WD- and Kelch-repeat proteins reveals particular functional classes that are common for both and other classes that are represented only by WD-repeat proteins but not Kelch-repeat proteins (Table 3).

Most prominent among the functional classes that are common between WD- and Kelch-repeat proteins are substrate adapters for ubiquitin E3 ligases. Ubiquitin E3 ligases mediate the conjugation of ubiquitin onto specific target proteins, typically to signal their destruction by the ubiquitin-proteasome pathway. Cullin Ring Ligases (CRLs) are a large class of E3 ligases that are assembled on a cullin scaffold protein. Cullin is an elongated protein that binds a substrate targeting adaptor protein at its N-terminus and a RING domain protein at its C-terminus.[42] The RING domain protein recruits the ubiquitin E2 enzyme that catalyzes the transfer of ubiquitin to a substrate bound by the substrate-targeting component. In animals, there are multiple cullin proteins and they associate with distinct classes of substrate targeting components.

CRLs assembled with Cullin1 (CUL1) use F-Box proteins as substrate targeting components; the N-terminal F-Box mediates the association with Cul1 via the Skp1 adaptor protein and the C-terminus of the F-Box protein contains a substrate-binding domain.[42] WD- and Kelch-repeat domains, among others, form the substrate binding domains for F-Box substrate adaptor proteins. Among the best characterized F-Box adaptor proteins are the WD-repeat proteins β-TrCP and Cdc4.[43] In addition, more than 20 additional F-Box/WD-repeat proteins are predicted in the human genome (Table 2) and these are likely to also function as CRL substrate adaptors.[42] In contrast, animal genomes appear to only contain one or two F-Box proteins with Kelch-repeat domains and these predicted proteins have not been characterized. Curiously, the prevalence of WD- and Kelch-repeat domains in *Arabidopsis* F-Box proteins is essentially the opposite as that in animal genomes. Only two F-Box proteins are paired with WD-repeat substrate binding domains,[33] but over 40 F-Box proteins have a C-terminal Kelch-repeat domain.[32,33] Several of these have been functionally characterized and are involved in degradation of circadian rhythm proteins.[44-46]

Cullin3 (CUL3) based E3 ligases use BTB proteins instead of F-Box proteins as substrate adaptors.[47,48] The BTB domain binds directly with Cullin3 and an additional domain mediates substrate targeting, the most common of which in vertebrates is the Kelch-repeat domain.[47] More than 40 genes encoding BTB-Kelch proteins have been identified in the human genome and most or all of these are likely to function as CUL3-associated substrate adaptor proteins. Thus far, no

Table 3. Representative functional classes of WD- and Kelch-repeat proteins

	WD	Kelch
E3 ligase substrate adapter	β-TrCP/Slimb, Cdc4p, Met30p, Sel10 ≥ 20 additional predicted in mammalian genomes	Keap1, Gigaxonin, KLHL9/KLHL13, KLHL10, Kelch ≥40 predicted in mammalian genomes ≥40 predicted in *Arabidopsis* genome
Cytoskeletal/Cell polarity	**Actin** Coronin family proteins Aip1p ARPC1 **Microtubule** LIS1 dynein IC katanin p80 **Cell Polarity** Lgl	Kelch, α-scruin, Mayven, ENC-1, IPP, Calicin, actin-fragmin kinase Kel1p, Kel2p (*S. cerevisiae*) Tea1p (*S. pombe*) Muskelin
Transcriptional regulation	TAFII Groucho/TLE Tup1p, Esc HIRA/CAF-1 p60 subunit	HCF
Signaling	G-β RACK1 Bub3 CDC20	Attractin/Mahagony
Vesicle trafficking	Coatomer subunits: α-COP, β-COP COPII coat subunits: Sec13p, Sec31p	p40
RNA processing	Sli8p CstF-50 Prp17 Prp4	

WD-repeat domains have been identified within BTB domain proteins (Table 2). The *Arabidopsis* genome, which appears to rely heavily on the Kelch-repeat domain as the substrate-binding domain in F-Box proteins, appears to contain only a few genes that contain a BTB domain paired with a Kelch-repeat domain.

The budding and fission yeast genomes contain only five F-Box/WD-repeat proteins and no BTB/Kelch proteins.[42] Most of the CRL substrate adaptors from higher eukaryotes that have been characterized have only one known substrate (e.g., Keap1) or target several distinct proteins through a similar recognition motif in several proteins (e.g., Cdc4p). It thus appears that the WD- and Kelch-repeat domain CRL families underwent expansion as the additional regulatory requirements associated with multicellular life emerged. Presumably, genes encoding WD- and Kelch-repeat domain CRL substrate adaptors underwent duplication and divergence to evolve new target specificities. The large number of WD- and Kelch-repeat domains in CRL substrate adaptors may be a consequence of their ability to rapidly evolve new binding affinities.

Another functional class of proteins containing many WD- and Kelch-repeat domains is cytoskeletal regulatory proteins (Table 3). WD-repeat domain proteins have diverse roles in regulating both the actin and microtubules. In some cases, the WD-domain makes direct contact with cytoskeletal filaments, as appears to be the case for the F-actin regulators of the Coronin-family[49,50] and ARPC1[37] and probably also Aip1p.[51] Each of these WD-domain proteins makes contacts with other cytoskeletal proteins as well; thus the WD-repeat regulators of the actin cytoskeleton may coordinate the action of multiple F-actin regulatory proteins. Similarly, WD-repeat proteins that regulate the microtubule cytoskeleton appear to function in conjunction with other microtubule interacting proteins. These include LIS1, which interacts with both dynein and proteins associated with the growing ends of microtubules[52] and the p80 subunit of the microtubule severing protein katanin.[53] Of note, the Coronin protein has also been reported to bind microtubules and so may represent a protein that regulates both of these filament systems simultaneously.[49] The common functional theme involves coordinating the action of cytoskeletal interacting proteins.

Most Kelch-repeat proteins involved in cytoskeletal regulation interact with F-actin. Indeed, a number of proteins, including *Drosophila* Kelch,[54] *Limulus* α-Scruin[55] and the mammalian proteins Mayven,[56] IPP,[57] ENC-1,[58] actin-fragmin kinase[59,60] and Calicin[61] have all been shown to bind F-actin, but interactions with other cytoskeletal regulatory proteins have not been reported. Interestingly, Kelch, Mayven, IPP and ENC1 all have N-terminal BTB domains, raising the question of whether these proteins also associate with CUL3 to form E3 CRLs. We have found that in *Drosophila*, Kelch does in fact associate with CUL3 and that loss of CUL3 leads to a similar phenotype as that of Kelch (AH and LC, manuscript in preparation). However, we have seen no evidence that actin is a target for ubiquitination by a Kelch/CUL3 CRL, so understanding the distinct functions of F-actin binding and ubiquitin substrate targeting will await further work. Tea1p is the one Kelch repeat protein that appears to regulate the microtubule cytoskeleton.[62] This protein contains N-terminal Kelch repeats and a C-terminal coiled-coil and is required for proper microtubule organization during polarized growth in *S. pombe*. Presently, it is not known whether Tea1p interacts directly with microtubules or microtubule regulatory proteins.

Functional groupings of WD- and Kelch-repeat proteins also reveal that WD-repeats are prominent in a number of functional classes where Kelch-repeats are poorly represented. The WD-repeat family contains a significant number of proteins involved in transcriptional regulation, RNA metabolism, vesicle trafficking and signal transduction; in contrast, there are few or no known examples of Kelch-repeat proteins that function in these pathways.

Conclusions

Recent advances on structures and functions of WD- and Kelch-repeat proteins have provided a better general understanding of these protein families. While folding into similar core structures, the active binding surfaces are distinct for the two classes of β-propellers. Variable surface loops are restricted to the top surface of Kelch-repeat β-propellers, while WD-repeat proteins have variable loops on both surfaces. This may explain some of the trends emerging from functional experiments. Kelch-repeat domains studied to date bind to only one partner and structural work on Keap1 suggests that this occurs on the top face of the propeller. In contrast, WD-repeats can have one or more binding partners, using binding sites on both the top and bottom of the β-propeller.

Acknowledgements

Our work on Kelch-related protiens is supported by NIH grant GM052702.

References

1. Neer E, Schmidt C, Nambudripad R et al. The ancient regulatory-protein family of WD-repeat proteins. Nature 1994; 371(6495):297-300.
2. Way M, Sanders M, Garcia C et al. Sequence and domain organization of scruin, an actin-cross-linking protein in the acrosomal process of Limulus sperm. J Cell Biol 1995; 128(1-2):51-60.
3. Xue F, Cooley L. kelch encodes a component of intercellular bridges in Drosophila egg chambers. Cell 1993; 72(5):681-693.
4. Li D, Roberts R. WD-repeat proteins: structure characteristics, biological function and their involvement in human diseases. Cell Mol Life Sci 2001; 58(14):2085-2097.

5. Smith T, Gaitatzes C, Saxena K et al. The WD repeat: a common architecture for diverse functions. Trends Biochem Sci 1999; 24(5):181-185.
6. Yu L, Gaitatzes C, Neer E et al. Thirty-plus functional families from a single motif. Protein Sci 2000; 9(12):2470-2476.
7. Adams J, Kelso R, Cooley L. The kelch repeat superfamily of proteins: propellers of cell function. Trends Cell Biol 2000; 10(1):17-24.
8. Prag S, Adams J. Molecular phylogeny of the kelch-repeat superfamily reveals an expansion of BTB/kelch proteins in animals. BMC Bioinformatics 2003; 4:42.
9. Madrona A, Wilson D. The structure of Ski8p, a protein regulating mRNA degradation: Implications for WD protein structure. Protein Sci 2004; 13(6):1557-1565.
10. Ito N, Phillips SE, Stevens C et al. Novel thioether bond revealed by a 1.7 A crystal structure of galactose oxidase. Nature 1991; 350(6313):87-90.
11. Lambright DG, Sondek J, Bohm A et al. The 2.0 A crystal structure of a heterotrimeric G protein. Nature 1996; 379(6563):311-319.
12. Sondek J, Bohm A, Lambright DG et al. Crystal structure of a G-protein beta gamma dimer at 2.1A resolution. Nature 1996; 379(6563):369-374.
13. Li X, Zhang D, Hannink M et al. Crystal structure of the Kelch domain of human Keap1. J Biol Chem 2004; 279(52):54750-54758.
14. Padmanabhan B, Tong K, Ohta T et al. Structural basis for defects of Keap1 activity provoked by its point mutations in lung cancer. Mol Cell 2006; 21(5):689-700.
15. Wall M, Coleman D, Lee E et al. The structure of the G protein heterotrimer Gi alpha 1 beta 1 gamma 2. Cell 1995; 83(6):1047-1058.
16. Beamer L, Li X, Bottoms C et al. Conserved solvent and side-chain interactions in the 1.35 Angstrom structure of the Kelch domain of Keap1. Acta Crystallogr D Biol Crystallogr 2005; 61(Pt 10):1335-1342.
17. Bork P, Doolittle R. Drosophila kelch motif is derived from a common enzyme fold. J Mol Biol 1994; 236(5):1277-1282.
18. Paoli M. Protein folds propelled by diversity. Prog Biophys Mol Biol 2001; 76(1-2):103-130.
19. Jawad-Alami Z, Paoli M. Novel sequences propel familiar folds. Structure 2002; 10(4):447-454.
20. Murzin A. Structural principles for the propeller assembly of beta-sheets: the preference for seven-fold symmetry. Proteins 1992; 14(2):191-201.
21. Beisel H, Kawabata S, Iwanaga S et al. Tachylectin-2: crystal structure of a specific GlcNAc/GalNAc-binding lectin involved in the innate immunity host defense of the Japanese horseshoe crab Tachypleus tridentatus. EMBO J 1999; 18(9):2313-2322.
22. Kiyosue T, Wada M. LKP1 (LOV kelch protein 1): a factor involved in the regulation of flowering time in arabidopsis. Plant J 2000; 23(6):807-815.
23. Nelson D, Lasswell J, Rogg L et al. FKF1, a clock-controlled gene that regulates the transition to flowering in Arabidopsis. Cell 2000; 101(3):331-340.
24. Somers DE, Schultz TF, Milnamow M et al. ZEITLUPE encodes a novel clock-associated PAS protein from Arabidopsis. Cell 2000; 101(3):319-329.
25. Finn RD, Mistry J, Schuster-Bockler B et al. Pfam: clans, web tools and services. Nucleic Acids Res 2006; 34(Database issue):D247-251.
26. Larsen N, Harrison S. Crystal structure of the spindle assembly checkpoint protein Bub3. J Mol Biol 2004; 344(4):885-892.
27. Voegtli W, Madrona A, Wilson D. The structure of Aip1p, a WD repeat protein that regulates Cofilin-mediated actin depolymerization. J Biol Chem 2003; 278(36):34373-34379.
28. Wilson D, Cerna D, Chew E. The 1.1-angstrom structure of the spindle checkpoint protein Bub3p reveals functional regions. J Biol Chem 2005; 280(14):13944-13951.
29. Orlicky S, Tang X, Willems A et al. Structural basis for phosphodependent substrate selection and orientation by the SCFCdc4 ubiquitin ligase. Cell 2003; 112(2):243-256.
30. Garcia-Higuera I, Gaitatzes C, Smith T et al. Folding a WD repeat propeller. Role of highly conserved aspartic acid residues in the G protein beta subunit and Sec13. J Biol Chem 1998; 273(15):9041-9049.
31. Owen C, DeRosier D. A 13-A map of the actin-scruin filament from the limulus acrosomal process. J Cell Biol 1993; 123(2):337-344.
32. Andrade M, González-Guzmán M, Serrano R et al. A combination of the F-box motif and kelch repeats defines a large Arabidopsis family of F-box proteins. Plant Mol Biol 2001; 46(5):603-614.
33. Kuroda H, Takahashi N, Shimada H et al. Classification and expression analysis of Arabidopsis F-box-containing protein genes. Plant Cell Physiol 2002; 43(10):1073-1085.
34. Jennings B, Pickles L, Wainwright S et al. Molecular recognition of transcriptional repressor motifs by the WD domain of the Groucho/TLE corepressor. Mol Cell 2006; 22(5):645-655.

35. Tarricone C, Perrina F, Monzani S et al. Coupling PAF signaling to dynein regulation: structure of LIS1 in complex with PAF-acetylhydrolase. Neuron 2004; 44(5):809-821.
36. Robinson R, Turbedsky K, Kaiser D et al. Crystal structure of Arp2/3 complex. Science 2001; 294(5547):1679-1684.
37. Beltzner C, Pollard T. Identification of functionally important residues of Arp2/3 complex by analysis of homology models from diverse species. J Mol Biol 2004; 336(2):551-565.
38. Lo S, Li X, Henzl M et al. Structure of the Keap1:Nrf2 interface provides mechanistic insight into Nrf2 signaling. EMBO J 2006; 25(15):3605-3617.
39. Cullinan SB, Gordan JD, Jin J et al. The Keap1-BTB protein is an adaptor that bridges Nrf2 to a Cul3-based E3 ligase: oxidative stress sensing by a Cul3-Keap1 ligase. Mol Cell Biol 2004; 24(19):8477-8486.
40. Kobayashi A, Kang MI, Okawa H et al. Oxidative stress sensor Keap1 functions as an adaptor for Cul3-based E3 ligase to regulate proteasomal degradation of Nrf2. Mol Cell Biol 2004; 24(16):7130-7139.
41. Zhang DD, Lo SC, Cross JV et al. Keap1 is a redox-regulated substrate adaptor protein for a Cul3-dependent ubiquitin ligase complex. Mol Cell Biol 2004; 24(24):10941-10953.
42. Petroski M, Deshaies R. Function and regulation of cullin-RING ubiquitin ligases. Nat Rev Mol Cell Biol 2005; 6(1):9-20.
43. Patton E, Willems A, Tyers M. Combinatorial control in ubiquitin-dependent proteolysis: don't Skp the F-box hypothesis. Trends Genet 1998; 14(6):236-243.
44. Han L, Mason M, Risseeuw E et al. Formation of an SCF(ZTL) complex is required for proper regulation of circadian timing. Plant J 2004; 40(2):291-301.
45. Imaizumi T, Schultz T, Harmon F et al. FKF1 F-box protein mediates cyclic degradation of a repressor of CONSTANS in Arabidopsis. Science 2005; 309(5732):293-297.
46. Sawa M, Nusinow D, Kay S et al. FKF1 and GIGANTEA Complex Formation is Required for Day-Length Measurement in Arabidopsis. Science 2007;318 (5848):261-265.
47. Stogios P, Downs G, Jauhal J et al. Sequence and structural analysis of BTB domain proteins. Genome Biol 2005; 6(10):R82.
48. Xu L, Wei Y, Reboul J et al. BTB proteins are substrate-specific adaptors in an SCF-like modular ubiquitin ligase containing CUL-3. Nature 2003; 425(6955):316-321.
49. Rybakin V, Clemen C. Coronin proteins as multifunctional regulators of the cytoskeleton and membrane trafficking. Bioessays 2005; 27(6):625-632.
50. Uetrecht A, Bear J. Coronins: the return of the crown. Trends Cell Biol 2006; 16(8):421-426.
51. Ono S. Regulation of actin filament dynamics by actin depolymerizing factor/cofilin and actin-interacting protein 1: new blades for twisted filaments. Biochemistry 2003; 42(46):13363-13370.
52. Xiang X. LIS1 at the microtubule plus end and its role in dynein-mediated nuclear migration. J Cell Biol 2003; 160(3):289-290.
53. McNally KP, Bazirgan OA, McNally FJ. Two domains of p80 katanin regulate microtubule severing and spindle pole targeting by p60 katanin. J Cell Sci 2000; 113(Pt 9):1623-1633.
54. Kelso R, Hudson A, Cooley L. Drosophila Kelch regulates actin organization via Src64-dependent tyrosine phosphorylation. J Cell Biol 2002; 156(4):703-713.
55. Sun S, Footer M, Matsudaira P. Modification of Cys-837 identifies an actin-binding site in the beta-propeller protein scruin. Mol Biol Cell 1997; 8(3):421-430.
56. Soltysik-Espanola M, Rogers RA, Jiang S et al. Characterization of Mayven, a novel actin-binding protein predominantly expressed in brain. Mol Biol Cell 1999; 10(7):2361-2375.
57. Kim IF, Mohammadi E, Huang RC. Isolation and characterization of IPP, a novel human gene encoding an actin-binding, kelch-like protein. Gene 1999; 228(1-2):73-83.
58. Hernandez MC, Andres-Barquin PJ, Martinez S et al. ENC-1: a novel mammalian kelch-related gene specifically expressed in the nervous system encodes an actin-binding protein. J Neurosci 1997; 17(9):3038-3051.
59. Eichinger L, Bomblies L, Vandekerckhove J et al. A novel type of protein kinase phosphorylates actin in the actin-fragmin complex. EMBO J 1996; 15(20):5547-5556.
60. Steinbacher S, Hof P, Eichinger L et al. The crystal structure of the Physarum polycephalum actin-fragmin kinase: an atypical protein kinase with a specialized substrate-binding domain. EMBO J 1999; 18(11):2923-2929.
61. Lecuyer C, Dacheux JL, Hermand E et al. Actin-binding properties and colocalization with actin during spermiogenesis of mammalian sperm calicin. Biol Reprod 2000; 63(6):1801-1810.
62. Mata J, Nurse P. tea1 and the microtubular cytoskeleton are important for generating global spatial order within the fission yeast cell. Cell 1997; 89(6):939-949.
63. The PyMOL Molecular Graphics System (http://www.pymol.org) [computer program]. Version 0.99: DeLano Scientific, Palo Alto, CA; 2002.

64. Nolen B, Pollard T. Insights into the influence of nucleotides on actin family proteins from seven structures of Arp2/3 complex. Mol Cell 2007; 26(3):449-457.
65. Wu G, Xu G, Schulman B et al. Structure of a beta-TrCP1-Skp1-beta-catenin complex: destruction motif binding and lysine specificity of the SCF(beta-TrCP1) ubiquitin ligase. Mol Cell 2003; 11(6):1445-1456.
66. Appleton B, Wu P, Wiesmann C. The crystal structure of murine coronin-1: a regulator of actin cytoskeletal dynamics in lymphocytes. Structure 2006; 14(1):87-96.
67. Pickles L, Roe S, Hemingway E et al. Crystal structure of the C-terminal WD40 repeat domain of the human Groucho/TLE1 transcriptional corepressor. Structure 2002; 10(6):751-761.
68. Cerna D, Wilson D. The structure of Sif2p, a WD repeat protein functioning in the SET3 corepressor complex. J Mol Biol 2005; 351(4):923-935.
69. Cheng Z, Liu Y, Wang C et al. Crystal structure of Ski8p, a WD-repeat protein with dual roles in mRNA metabolism and meiotic recombination. Protein Sci 2004; 13(10):2673-2684.
70. Sprague E, Redd M, Johnson A et al. Structure of the C-terminal domain of Tup1, a corepressor of transcription in yeast. EMBO J 2000; 19(12):3016-3027.

Chapter 2

Diversity of WD-Repeat Proteins

Temple F. Smith*

Abstract

The WD-repeat-containing proteins form a very large family that is diverse in both its function and domain structure. Within all these proteins the WD-repeat domains are thought to have two common features: the domain folds into a beta propeller; and the domains form a platform without any catalytic activity on which multiple protein complexes assemble reversibly. The fact that these proteins play such key roles in the formation of protein-protein complexes in nearly all the major pathways and organelles unique to eukaryotic cells has two important implications. It supports both their ancient and proto eukaryotic origins and supports a likely association with many genetic diseases.

Introduction

Many protein families are characterized by their common sequence motifs, catalytic function and/or structure. WD-repeat domain-containing proteins comprise one such family characterized by a common sequence repeat named for the high frequency of the tryptophan and aspartic acid pairs that generally define the end of its approximately 40-residue-long amino acids. While the sequence repeat contains no absolutely conserved positions, the basic pattern is well-conserved (see Fig. 1A). Structurally the domains containing these repeats belong to the larger class of proteins having the beta propeller fold. These are highly symmetric folds composed of between four and eight anti-parallel, four-stranded beta sheets arranged radially around a central axis, as shown in Figure 1B. In the case of the WD-repeat-containing proteins, each WD repeat is part of one of the four anti-parallel strands that form one of the "blades" of these propeller-like structures. The full WD sequence-repeat is not equivalent to a single blade, but rather each contains the first three strands of one blade and the fourth of the adjacent blade. While beta propeller structures are found throughout both Prokaryota and Eukaryota, the WD-repeat beta propellers are found primarily among eukaryotes.[1]

There is no common function within the larger protein structural family of the beta propellers, as is true for most families defined only by their common fold. At one level this is also true within the WD sequence repeat family, where there is no common function in terms of substrate binding, catalytic activity or pathway membership. What does appear to be the common feature is the ability of that domain to interact reversibly with multiple other proteins to form complexes.[2] It forms a stable platform or scaffold on which large protein-protein complexes assemble. This WD-repeat-containing domain is found throughout Eukaryota, ranging from a few to over a hundred distinct proteins in mammals. It functions in signal transduction, RNA processing, vesicular trafficking, cytoskeleton assembly, cell cycle regulation, transcription of the initiation complex and many other processes (see Table 1).

Figure 1B,C displays a typical WD-repeat protein, beta-TrCP1 ubiquitin ligase. This protein is a multidomain protein containing both a WD and an F-box domain (mediates interaction

*Temple F. Smith—BioMolecular Engineering Research Center, College of Engineering, Boston University, 36 Cummington Street, Boston, MA 02215, USA. Email: tsmith@darwin.bu.edu

The Coronin Family of Proteins, edited by Christoph S. Clemen, Ludwig Eichinger and Vasily Rybakin. ©2008 Landes Bioscience and Springer Science+Business Media.

Table 1. A partial list of cellular pathways and functions involving WD-repeat-containing proteins

Pathway/Function	Example Genes
G-protein signal transduction	Gbb/FYVE
RNA processing and splicing	SOF1/PRP4/PRP19
tRNA and 60s rRNA processing	Rsa40
Translation initiation complex formation	TFIID
Chromatin assembly, histone acetylation	CAF1/RpaP/MSI1
Polyadenylation in polymerase II transcription termination	RAE1/Swd2
Vesicular trafficking	NORI-1/WDR1
Golgi trafficking	SEC13
Cilia assemble	IC138/IC140I/FTA-1
Mitochondria division control	Mdv1p
Platelet activation	LIS1
Lymphocyte homing	WAIT-1
Phagocytosis/actin binding	CRN/CORO/p57
Cytoskeleton/myosin assembly	MHCK-A/B/C
Photomorphogenesis, in higher plants	SPA-quartet
Ribosomal assembly and intra-nuclear transport	Rsa4p
Regulation of cell cycle progression	CDC40/Pop1/Pop2
Cell division/chromatin separation	HIR
Cell/tissue differentiation	hag/Wdr1
Gene transcription activation and corepression	Hir1p
Targeting associated catalytic domains	
Kinases	MHCK-A/B/C
Ubiquitin degradation	Ufd3p
Phospholipase activation	DOA1/PLAP

with Skp1 linking F-box proteins to a ubiquitin-ligase complex). It, like many WD-repeat proteins, contains both an insert within the WD-repeat domain forming an additional small structure on one of the domain's surfaces and is multidomained. The F-box WD-repeat combination proteins form a rather large family. This includes Pop1 and Pop2 proteins, which in yeast play a key role in cell cycle progression.[3]

Perhaps the best studied member of this family is the beta subunit of the trimeric G-protein, a key signal transduction system found throughout Eukaryota.[4] In this case, nearly the entire beta subunit consists of seven WD sequence repeats that form a seven-bladed beta propeller.[5-7] In addition there is a short alpha helical domain at the C-terminal end that binds nearly irreversibly to the gamma subunit (composed of only two alpha helices). One additional curious fact is that at least in the case of *Dictyostelium*, this G-beta-gamma combination requires an additional protein, PhLP1[8] for assembly. This beta-gamma G-protein subunit interacts with the catalytic alpha subunit in its inactive receptor bound state. The activation of the G-protein receptor catalyzes the exchange of GDP in the alpha subunit for GTP. That in turn causes the separate release from the receptor of the G-beta-gamma subunit and the G-alpha subunit. Both then interact reversibly with a number of other downstream proteins within various signaling cascades.[9-12]

The Beta Propeller Structure

This common fold variously contains from four to nine anti-parallel four-stranded beta sheets.[1] These are arrayed radially with a geometry similar to a ship's propeller, each propeller blade being composed of four anti-parallel strands, each slightly twisted in the same orientation. The height or length of the strands within each blade is near constant within a given protein, but can vary over a rather wide range from a minimum of four to 10 amino acids in different proteins. These structures define three surfaces, a circular top and bottom and a cylindrical circumference. In many cases part of the cylindrical surface is in contact with one or more additional domains that are part of the same protein. For example, in the above noted trimeric G-protein beta subunit, there is the short helical domain contacting part of both the cylindrical and the bottom surfaces. In the archaeal surface layer beta propeller protein, SLP,[13] there are multiple copies of a second all-beta domain making extensive surface contacts with the beta propeller domain. The latter protein is a particularly interesting example. It, like the G-protein WD beta subunit, forms a seven-bladed propeller and contains a sequence repeat with a distinctive YVTN amino acid motif. This protein in fact contains two very similar seven-bladed beta propellers and 12 repeated small all-beta domains (see Fig. 3 in Jing et al 2002).[13] In addition, it shows similarity to a metazoan cell surface set of seven-bladed beta propeller protein receptors that contain the YWTD motif.[13] The similarity in both cellular location and sequence motif suggests a potential common origin of these proteins. As discussed below, however, there is no such similar example to guide us in attempting to identify the ancestor of the eukaryotic WD-repeat proteins. Kostlanova et al[14] identified a beta propeller from *Ralstonia solanacearum* formed by oligomerization rather than being contained within a single peptide as are other known beta propeller proteins, including all known WD-repeat domains.

There are other beta propeller families with very similar fold structures to the WD-repeat family, such as the EAR domain family. These form seven-bladed propellers with amino acid repeats averaging 44 residues long.[15] Interestingly they have a weakly conserved sequence motif that includes a tryptophan polar amino acid pair at the end of the fourth strand, as compared to the tryptophan aspartic acid pair common to the end of the third strand in the WD-repeat family. Also like the WD-repeat domain, the EAR domain generally occurs within a larger multidomain protein. One structural fact about the WD-repeat beta propellers and other beta propeller families is that the amino acid composition internal to the region of beta sheet-to-sheet contacts does not vary as a function of the number of repeats. Thus as the overall size increases, from four to more blades, any needed change in the side chain packing is compensated by slight changes in blade twist and side chain rotomers. This again seems to support the idea of a very stable fold configuration for these proteins. However as seen in Figure 1B, the WD-repeat proteins close their propeller circular structures with a Velcro-like overlap of the third strand of the last blade with an outer strand from the first of the WD repeats. Many nonWD propellers do not use this closure method. For example the YWTD motif-containing propellers form all blades sequentially, each containing the complete sequence repeat.

The Identification of WD Repeats

Given the variation in size, composition, function and domain structure the accurate identification of all WD-repeat-containing proteins has been a challenge. As an example, the distribution of WD-repeat-containing proteins in plants has been investigated in the model system, *Arabidopsis*, by van Nocker and Ludwig.[16,17] They identified 237 potential WD-repeat-containing proteins falling into what they believed to be more than 50 distinct families. Their approach involved identifying all *Arabidopsis* proteins containing at least four WD-repeat patterns as defined by patterns and/or examples in Prosite, Pfam, PRINTS and SMART.[18] These were then clustered using Blastclust (http://www.NCBI.nlm.nih.gov). This is a rather straightforward general approach, similar to that employed by the BioMolecular Engineering Research Center at Boston University, which maintains the WD-repeat database (on the web at http://bmerc.bu.edu). The basic sequence repeat can be identified as a weakly conserved motif, as shown in Figure 1A, with an overall sequence compatibility with a probable structure.

The difficulty in identifying members of WD-repeat families is two-fold: first the pattern is not absolutely conserved, even in part; and second, in any standard sequence comparison search, the different repeats in a given protein will match many WD repeats in a wide range of different family representatives over a very wide range of statistical significance. The variation in the number of blades within different subfamilies of WD-repeat proteins and the fact that different WD-repeat families often contain at least one of the same additional domains, makes subfamily distinction difficult. This difficulty can be acute and is compounded by the fact that WD-repeat proteins often have one or more such nonWD domains inserted within and between the WD repeats that form a single beta propeller (see Fig. 1B,C).

The seven-bladed propeller structure of the coronin family contains only five clearly identifiable WD repeats. These WD repeats are found between positions 79 and 305 in the murine coronin 1 (coronin 1A).[19] The first and last blades, 37-71 and 306-352 are either very highly modified WD repeats or were derived from a different source. While it is possible that five WD repeats were inserted into some pre-existing beta domain, this seems a bit unlikely given the standard Velcro-type propeller closure is employed. In addition the strand order in these two non WD repeats is the same as that in the five WD repeats. It is clear that the sequences of these two non WD repeats are by themselves diagnostic of the coronin family.

There is a curious and characteristic feature of the WD-repeat domains. This is that the most conserved position for a particular amino acid in the WD repeat is not in the "defining" trp/asp pair at the end of the third strand, but an aspartic acid in the turn between the second and third strand of each propeller blade. This amino acid position effectively forms a highly polar, normally negative charged ring on the top of the propeller. A second feature containing a very limited range of amino acids (see Fig. 1A) is the run of three small side chain amino acids at the C-terminal end of the second blade's strand. Finally there is the turn/loop region between strands 1 and 2, which while often varying in length, generally contains a proline aspartic acid or aspartate glycine classic reverse turn. Such distinctive features often allow the identification of the WD repeat even when other features are either missing or weak.

The above considerations require an iterative approach in which one first identifies all highly probable WD repeats within each protein of interest. Next one attempts to examine the rest of the protein for more divergent repeats that have the expected length and fall in the neighborhood or between clear WD repeats. In addition the sequence must be examined for other domains that may interrupt the sequence of WD repeats, but are known to occur in some WD families. Finally there must be a reasonable probability that there are at least four WD repeats, as no beta propeller is stable with fewer than four blades. There is also the likelihood that this structure is limited to no more than nine blades, as the central axis would be open to the solvent, reducing its stability. Under the assumption that it is the WD-repeat domain's surfaces that primarily define its role in protein-protein interactions, common features among the surface amino acids should be useful in identifying members of any given WD-repeat subfamily.

There are numerous sequence pattern tools to carry out the initial step above. There is, however, no single obvious approach for the remaining steps. One useful approach is the use of a set of probabilistic Hidden Markov Models.[20] Such models allow one to assign probabilities or likelihoods to the WD-repeat pattern elements individually, to the total number of such repeats, to their length ranges and to the chance and lengths of likely inserted non WD-repeat domains (see schematic in Fig. 1B,C). The probabilities used in such an HMM are determined either by observational experience using protein expert knowledge to anticipate yet unseen variations,[20] or by computational model training algorithms[21] on sets of known examples. In any case while a very large number of WD-repeat proteins can be straightforwardly recognized, there are undoubtedly both false positives and missed examples in both the literature and the annotated databases. Thus there is some uncertainty within the representative species distribution statistics given in Table 2.

While the WD-repeat proteins are rare in Prokaryota, there have been five identified among the 500-plus sequenced bacterial genomes, for example, the noncanonical WD-repeats of Hat found in the cyanobacterium *Synechocystis*.[22] This protein is involved in inorganic carbon transport and has five significant repeats matching the pattern shown in Figure 1A. It also has five or six additional weaker repeats with the potential for a total of eleven.

The Functions Carried Out by the WD-Repeat Family

These proteins are involved in a very wide range of cellular functions. In all cases studied in detail, the actual beta propeller WD-repeat domain is not involved in any catalytic function. This is in contrast to many beta propeller, nonWD-repeat domains, as in the case of the fructosyl transferases.[23] As noted above, the WD-repeat domains provide multiple protein-protein binding surfaces for reversible protein complex formation.[2] A particularly interesting example has been seen in the East African cichlid fishes, the *hag* gene.[24] This is a member of the large class of the F-Box joint WD-repeat family known to regulate differentiation in the fly.[25] What was observed in the cichlid fish was a very rapid speciation correlated with accelerated surface amino acid selected changes on the

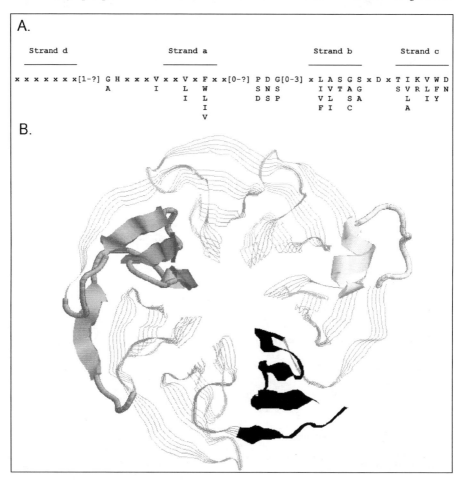

Figure 1. The beta WD propeller. A) The repeat-defining sequence's most common amino acids. "x" indicates any amino acid. Number in brackets indicate the known variable range. B) The F-box WD-repeat protein 1p22.pdb (beta-TrCP1) with dark gray strand cartoons defining the extent of a full WD-repeat. Shown in light gray alpha helix cartoon is an inserted loop between two WD-repeats. In black are three strands of the C-terminal blade overlapped by a first strand formed from the N-terminal end of the WD-repeat domain. In black is the Velcro last strand overlapped by the first strand of the first repeat. C) Displays an edge-on view of the WD repeat and the F-box domain extending above the upper surface of the propeller. Also shown in atomic space fill is the repeat-defining Trp-Asp pair.

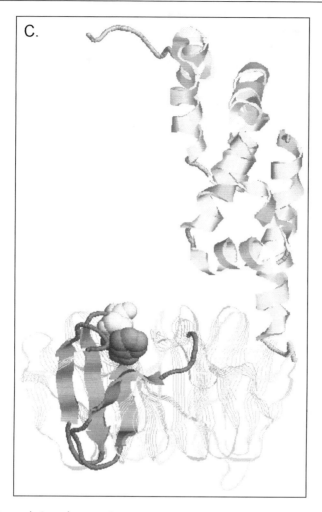

Figure 1C. Legend viewed on previous page.

WD-repeat domain. This clearly suggests that some of the speciation defining genetic events could be seen in the selective adaptation within these interacting surfaces effecting changes in pigment pattern.[24] The WD-repeat-containing protein, Wdr5[26] also plays a key role in differentiation, in this case that of osteoblasts and chondrocytes. There are a number of other well-studied examples of these surface protein-protein interactions[11,12] directly observed for various WD-repeat-containing proteins. These include the TFDII, required for transcription initiation complex formation and the IC138 and IC140 WD-repeat proteins required for dynein inner-arm motor complex formation in eukaryotic cilia.[27] A third WD-repeat protein, IFTA-1, is also involved in cilia assembly, in this case for the retrograde intraflagellar protein transport.[28] Identified in *Dictyostelium* is another WD protein, MHCK, which is involved with another motor protein, myosin. Here the WD-domain targets the myosin heavy chain kinases by binding to the myosin filaments.[29] One very well-studied WD-repeat protein is Lis1, a protein that regulates the microtubule motor cytoplasmic dynein, while in the vertebrate brain it is associated with the cytosolic PAF-acetylhydrolase. This interaction

Table 2. Distribution of WD-repeat counts in WD proteins among a set of representative eukaryotic species. The number pairs are the total probable WD proteins with a given range of repeats. In parentheses is the subset of those that contain at least one significant additional non WD domain

Species (Common Name)	Number of Repeats				
	4-6	7	8	9	>10
a. thaliana (thale cress weed)	12 (12)	111 (102)	57 (47)	16 (14)	22 (22)
m. domestica (plums)	12 (12)	94 (92)	54 (49)	13 (13)	31 (31)
s. cerevisiae (baker's yeast)	5 (5)	27 (26)	16 (13)	1 (1)	7 (7)
s. pombe (fission yeast)	4 (4)	42 (42)	19 (15)	5 (5)	7 (7)
s. purpuratus (purple sea urchin)	19 (19)	121 (108)	71 (65)	15 (15)	50 (50)
x. laevis (African clawed frog)	19 (19)	163 (158)	116 (94)	22 (22)	34 (34)
x. tropicalis (pipid frog)	15 (15)	103 (100)	75 (54)	12 (12)	26 (26)
d. melanogaster (fruit fly)	7 (7)	87 (86)	67 (61)	3 (3)	18 (18)
d. rerio (zebrafish)	18 (15)	94 (90)	50 (43)	11 (11)	25 (25)
m. musculus (mouse)	9 (8)	98 (97)	66 (58)	18 (18)	44 (44)
r. norvegicus (brown rat)	14 (14)	114 (113)	62 (53)	25 (25)	46 (46)
p. troglodytes (chimpanzee)	14 (14)	120 (119)	105 (101)	14 (13)	32 (32)
h. sapiens (human)	10 (9)	106 (104)	74 (66)	15 (15)	33 (33)

has been studied in a high resolution crystal structure revealing major protein-protein contacts with the upper circular surface of the WD domain.[30]

There is a WD yeast protein, Swd2, that plays an essential role in two distinct complex assemblies, the assembly of the peptide cleavage and polyadenylation factor and that of the lysine methylation of histone H3 complex.[31] More typical is the yeast protein, Mdv1p, that plays a key role in the assembly of a single complex, the mitochondrial division, Dnm1p, complex in conjunction with the mitochondrial outer membrane protein Fis1P.[32] In *Arabidopsis* the SPA1 protein is involved in phytochrome A-signal transduction complex[33] and is an example of a WD-repeat domain attached to a catalytic domain, in this case a kinase domain. There is a pair of WD-repeat proteins, Mad2 and BubR1, that together yield the kinetochore complex, involved in interaction with a histone deacetylase.[34] The complex appears capable of delaying anaphase by inhibiting ubiquitin ligation.

The Gemin5 WD-repeat protein interacts with at least five of the snRNP core proteins in forming the SMN complex.[35] This is a large protein with 13 predicted WD repeats and a C-terminal coiled-coil domain. The coiled-coil domain, like the WD itself, is a protein-protein interaction domain. The large number of WD repeats in Gemin5 suggests that there are probably two WD domains, one of seven repeats and a second of six or seven repeats. The probability of three protein-protein interaction domains creates the possibility of forming a very large heteromeric complex or of being capable of forming multiple but distinct ones. There are other WD-repeat proteins that contain additional protein-protein interaction domains. Three of these are found in the brain and are members of the striatin family containing a coiled-coil domain and calmodulin-binding domain[36] in addition to a WD domain. Two of these are expressed in the central nervous system and are somehow involved in dendrite growth while another, SG2NA, is expressed in both brain and muscle. All three are both cytosolic and membrane-bound.[36] Another WD-repeat protein, NDRP, is associated with neurons and is expressed in developing and regenerating neurons, particularly those of the olfactory epithelia and retina.[37]

The GRWD1, a large protein containing a glutamate-rich domain and four WD-repeats, with a second WD-repeat protein, Bop1, is part of the preribosomal complex in ribosomal biogenesis.[38] A WD-repeat protein with a related function is the Ras4p, which along with being required for 60S ribosomal transport is required for tRNA processing. As a final example, the SIF2 WD-repeat yeast protein containing an eight-bladed WD propeller[39] is key to the assembly of the Set3 complex. This complex is the histone deacetylase complex and a meiosis-specific repressor of sporulation genes. It is worthy of note that the top surface of this protein is highly conserved. A second domain in the SIF2 protein mediates its tetramerization and its eight-bladed propeller structure is distinct as a corepressor as compared to other corepressor families such as the Groucho WD-repeat family.[40] This WD protein plays an extensive role in gene expression associated with developmental patterning.[41] While the Groucho proteins do not bind DNA directly they appear to bind other proteins that do. The role of WD-repeat proteins in both animal and plant embryo patterning and development is well documented. For example the Xbub3 protein is distributed throughout the oocyte in the early stages and then gradually localized to the animal hemisphere in the perinuclear cytoplasm of mature oocytes.[42] While in the plant *Arabidopsis* the WD-repeat protein, TAN, has been shown to be required of embryo development via its interactions with other proteins.[43]

In a short review of the Human WD-repeat proteins Li and Roberts[44] noted their association with a number of human diseases. Some WD-repeat family proteins have been directly implicated in a particular human disease. For example the G-protein beta-3 subunit appears to have a splice variant that is causal in essential hypertension.[45] The Triple-A syndrome has been shown to be caused by mutations in the WD-repeat protein, AAAS.[46] The WD-repeat protein WAIT-1 is known to interact with the beta-7 integrins and affects lymphocyte homing in the normal immune response[47] and its mutation can disrupt that part of the immune response. The WD-repeat protein STRAP has an oncogenic affect in human carcinogenesis apparently through its interaction with transforming growth factor, TGF-beta.[48] The WD-repeat protein, endonulein, as a cell cycle protein is an oncogene for adenocarcinoma of the pancreas when up-regulated.[49] The human WDR11 protein is associated with glioblastoma via a chromosome translocation truncating the WD-repeat domain after the second of six repeats.[50] The Groucho family, which is key in developmental patterning as an organizer of gene repression, may play a role in colorectal cancer suppression via the Wnt signaling pathway.[51] There is a set of mutations in the WD-repeat domain of AHI1 that is associated with the autosomal recessive disorder, Houbert syndrome, involving mental retardation.[52] While this is only a short list of examples of WD domain disease correlations, the current functional list (in Table 1) of WD-repeat domain-containing protein functions is suggestive of a much wider range of potential inherited-disease associations.

There are of course many other functional complexes containing or organized by WD-repeat domains. Many of these involve signal transduction, the best studied being the large number of known trimeric G-proteins and their downstream complexes generally involving MAP Kinase cascades. Table 1 contains a list of these and other cellular functions, roles and/or pathways in which at least one WD-repeat-containing protein has been clearly shown. Included of course are the members of the actin binding family of coronin proteins discussed throughout the following chapters.

The Distribution and Origin of the Family

Table 2 lists the number of WD-repeat protein sequences identified with high confidence within various taxonomic divisions for particular species representatives. The numbers were obtained using simple sequence pattern recognition tools followed by a full-length protein sequence context analysis. They are presented in terms of the number of probable WD repeats and whether or not they contain additional domains of significant length.

The limited occurrences of WD repeats in the prokaryotic taxa raise the issue as to whether this family is of very ancient origin or, as has been suggested, is a eukaryotic invention borrowed by some prokaryotes via horizontal gene transfer. Given the very wide range in sequence, blade number and functions found among the beta propellers, one might wonder if they all had a common early ancestor. Or is it more likely that this fold is so naturally stable that nearly any four-fold plus repeat with high beta propensity of 36 to 50 amino acids will form this type of structure? Repeats at the DNA level are common mutational fare in all organisms. The possible eukaryotic origin is supported by the fact that so many of the WD-repeat proteins are involved in forms of signal transduction pathways unique to the eukaryotes. In addition few of the prokaryotic WD-repeat domain-containing protein examples have clear homologs in other prokaryotes. Also given the domain's ability to form large complexes, it could easily find utility if taken up by a prokaryote. Yet the potential homology of the archaeal surface layer protein (SLP)[13] YVTN-repeat seven-bladed beta propeller and the metazoan cell surface YWTD-repeat seven-bladed beta propeller cell surface receptors[13] supports a common ancestral relationship between these prokaryotic and eukaryotic protein families.

Most attempts at standard sequence phylogenetic analyses are difficult and/or inconclusive due to the high similarity within the structure-determining features of the WD repeats, overwhelming the functional family surface characteristics. By masking the beta propeller's internal repeat residues and then clustering only on the basis of the remaining sequence, there has been some success in functional grouping of the WD-repeat proteins. For example, surface analysis of one pair of proteins, MSI1 and Rb48 clustered them in the same subfamily, while the entire WD-repeat domain did not.[2] This clustering was verified by their partial complementation in yeast. Yet this did not allow any clear evolutionary relationships to emerge among these clustered functional subfamilies. Given that repeats are common in most beta propeller families of between four and eight blades, gene region expansion by duplication and contraction by deletion appears to have occurred many times. The fact that there are so many distinct repeat encoding beta propellers supports such a simple common genetic mechanistic origin. Yet given that these structures require at least four blades, one must also assume that some of these distinct families could have arisen through oligomerization as homo-tetramers or -dimers, as seen in *Ralstonia solanacearum*.[14]

Once a repeat is discovered to form a stable protein propeller platform, the sequence repeats can apparently be maintained and recognizable over a very long evolutionary period. There clearly has been functional selection on the surface residues and as to what additional domains are linked. On the other hand, negative or conserving selection appears to have been restricted to internal blade-to-blade packing, at least among this very large and diverse WD-repeat family. Given this variation in conserved repeats within, but not between, families, most repetitive beta propeller families seem likely to have independent origins. As for the origin of the WD-repeat superfamily, little is known. Without considerably more detailed information on the functions of the limited number of WD-repeat proteins found in prokaryotes one can only guess that the WD-repeat family is likely of eukaryotic origin. That of course would require that their occurrence in Prokaryota was probably the result of one or more horizontal gene transfer events. The issue is one of their distributional ubiquity in all Eukaryota, including components of so many unique eukaryotic functions, compared to limited and noncommon functions among the prokaryotes. While the eukaryotic WD-repeat families do seem to have the common function of protein-protein binding and complex assemblies, which if any of these was the first is very unclear. Signal transduction via the trimeric G-proteins of course is a possibility, but so is the essential role in RNA processing, in cilia or cytoskeleton assembly and in the initiation of transcription, all of which have been suggested as components of the last common ancestor of all extant eukaryotes. What is clear is that once this protein complex assembly aid was discovered, it was rapidly exploited throughout the earliest eukaryotes.

References
1. Paoli M. Protein folds propelled by diversity. Prog Biophys Mol Biol 2001; 76(1-2):103-30.
2. Smith TF, Gaitatzes C, Saxena K et al. The WD repeat: a common architecture for diverse functions. Trends Biochem Sci 1999; 24(5):181-85.
3. Kominami K, Ochotorena I, Toda T. Two F-box WD-repeat proteins Pop1 and Pop2 form hetero- and homo-complexes together with cullin-1 in the fission yeast SCF (Skp1-Cullin-1-F-box) ubiquitin ligase. Genes Cells 1998; 3:721-35.
4. Neer EJ. Heterotrimeric G-Proteins—Organizers of Transmembrane Signals. Cell 1995; 80(2):249-57.
5. Lambright DG, Sondek J, Bohm A et al. The 2.0 angstrom crystal structure of a heterotrimeric G protein. Nature 1996; 379(6563):311-19.
6. Neer EJ, Smith TF. G protein heterodimers: New structures propel new questions. Cell 1996; 84(2):175-78.
7. Wall MA, Coleman DE, Lee E et al. The Structure of the G-Protein Heterotrimer G(I-Alpha-1)Beta(1)Gamma(2). Cell 1995; 83(6):1047-58.
8. Knol JC, Engel R, Blaauw M et al. The Phosducin-Like Protein PhLP1 Is Essential for Gß Dimer Formation in Dictyostelium discoideum. Mol Cell Biol 2005; 25(18):8393-400.
9. Cabrera-Vera TM, Vanhauwe J, Thomas TO et al. Insights into G protein structure, function and regulation. Endocr Rev 2003; 24(6):765-81.
10. Katanaev VL, Tomlinson A. Dual roles for the trimeric G protein Go in asymmetric cell division in Drosophila. Proc Natl Acad Sci USA 2006; 103(17):6524-29.
11. Li Y, Sternweis PM, Charnecki S et al. Sites for G binding on the G protein subunit overlap with sites for regulation of Phospholipase C and Adenylyl. Cyclase J Biol Chem 1998; 273:16265-72.
12. Panchenko MP, Saxena K, Li Y et al. Sites important for PLC beta(2) activation by the G protein beta gamma subunit map to the sides of the beta propeller structure. J Biol Chem 1998; 273(43):28298-304.
13. Jing H, Takagi J, Liu JH et al. Archaeal surface layer proteins contain beta propeller, PKD and beta helix domains and are related to metazoan cell surface proteins. Structure 2002; 10(10):1453-64.
14. Kostlanova N, Mitchell EP, Lortat-Jacob H et al. The fucose-binding lectin from Ralstonia Solanacearum: a new type of beta-propeller architecture formed by oligomerisation and interacting with fucoside, fucosyllactose and plant xyloglucan. J Biol Chem 2005; 280(30):27839-27849.
15. Scheel H, Tomiuk S, Hofmann K. A common protein interaction domain links two recently identified epilepsy genes. Hum Mol Genet 2002; 11(15):1757-62.
16. van Nocker S, Ludwig P. The WD-repeat protein superfamily in Arabidopsis: conservation and divergence in structure and function. BMC Genomics 2003;4:50.
17. Zhong R, Ye Z-H. Molecular and Biochemical Characterization of Three WD-Repeat-Domain-containing Inositol Polyphosphate 5-Phosphatases in Arabidopsis thaliana. Plant Cell Physiol 2004; 45(11):1720-28.
18. Mulder NJ, Apweiler R, Attwood TK et al. The InterPro Database, 2003 brings increased coverage and new features. Nucleic Acids Res 2003; 31(1):315-18.
19. Appleton BA, Wu P, Wiesmann C. The crystal structure of murine coronin-1. Structure 2006; 14:87-89.
20. Yu L, Gaitatzes C, Neer EJ et al. Thirty-plus functional families from a single motif. Protein Sci 2000; 9:2470-76.
21. Hisbergues M, Gaitatzes CG, Joset F et al. A noncanonical WD-repeat protein from the cyanobacterium Synechocystis PCC6803: Structural and functional study. Protein Sci 2001; 10(2):293-300.
22. Rabiner LR. A Tutorial on Hidden Markov-Models and Selected Applications in Speech Recognition. Proc IEEE 1989; 77(2):257-86.
23. Pons T, Hernandez L, Batista FR et al. Prediction of a common beta-propeller catalytic domain for fructosyltranferases of different origin and substrate specificity. Protein Sci 2000; 9:2285-91.
24. Terai Y, Morikawa N, Kawakami K et al. Accelerated evolution of the surface amino acids in the WD-repeat domain encoded by the hagoromo gene in an explosively speciated lineage of east African cichlid fishes. Mol Biol Evol 2002; 19(4):574-78.
25. Jiang J, Struhl G. Regulation of the Hedgehog and Wingless signalling pathways by the F-box/WD40-repeat protein Slimb. Nature 1998; 391:493-96.
26. Gori F, Friedman L, Demay M. Wdr5, a novel WD repeat protein, regulates osteoblast and chondrocyte differentiation in vivo. J Musculoskelet Neuronal Interact 2005; 5(4):338-39.
27. Hendrickson TW, Perrone CA, Griffin P et al. IC138 is a WD-repeat dynein intermediate chain required for light chain assembly and regulation of flagellar bending. Mol Biol Cell 2004; 15(12):5431-42.

28. Blacque OE, Li C, Inglis PN et al. The WD Repeat-containing Protein IFTA-1 Is Required for Retrograde Intraflagellar Transport. MBC 2006; 17(12):5053-62.
29. Steimle PA, Naismith T, Licate L et al. WD repeat domains target Dictyostelium myosin heavy chain kinases by binding directly to myosin filaments. J Biol Chem 2001; 276(9):6853-60.
30. Tarricone C, Perrina F, Monzani S et al. Coupling PAF signaling to dynein regulation structure of LIS1 in complex with PAF-Acetylhydrolase. Neuron 2004; 44(5):809-21.
31. Cheng HL, He XY, Moore C. The essential WD repeat protein Swd2 has dual functions in RNA polymerase II transcription termination and lysine 4 methylation of histone H3. Mol Cell Biol 2004; 24(7):2932-43.
32. Tieu Q, Okreglak V, Naylor K et al. The WD repeat protein, Mdv1p, functions as a molecular adaptor by interacting with Dnm1p and Fis1p during mitochondrial fission. J Cell Biol 2002; 158(3):445-52.
33. Hoecker U, Tepperman JM, Quail PH. SPA1, a WD-repeat protein specific to phytochrome A signal transduction. Science 1999; 284(5413):496-99.
34. Yoon Y, Baek K, Jeong S et al. WD repeat-containing mitotic checkpoint proteins act as transcriptional repressors during interphase. FEBS Lett 2004; 575(1-3):23-29.
35. Gubitz AK, Mourelatos Z, Abel L et al. Gemin5, a novel WD repeat protein component of the SMN complex that binds Sm proteins. J Biol Chem 2002; 277(7):5631-36.
36. Castets F, Rakitina T, Gaillard S et al. Zinedin, SG2NA and striatin are calmodulin-binding, WD repeat proteins principally expressed in the brain. J Biol Chem 2000; 275(26):19970-77.
37. Kato H, Chen S, Kiyama H et al. Identification of a novel WD repeat—containing gene predominantly expressed in developing and regenerating neuron. J Biochem 2000; 128:923-32.
38. Gratenstein K, Heggestad AD, Fortun J et al. The WD-repeat protein GRWD1: Potential roles in myeloid differentiation and ribosome biogenesis. Genomics 2005; 85(6):762-73.
39. Cerna D, Wilson DK. The structure of sif2p, a WD repeat protein functioning in the SET3 corepressor complex. J Mol Biol 2005; 351(4):923-35.
40. Chen GQ, Courey AJ. Groucho/TLE family proteins and transcriptional repression. Gene 2000; 249(1-2):1-16.
41. Song HY, Hasson P, Paroush Z et al. Groucho oligomerization is required for repression in vivo. Mol Cell Biol 2004; 24(10):4341-50.
42. Goto T, Kinoshita T. Maternal transcripts of mitotic checkpoint gene, Xbub3, are accumulated in the animal blastomeres of Xenopus early embryo. DNA Cell Biol 1999; 18(3):227-34.
43. Yamagishi K, Nagata N, Yee KM et al. TANMEI/EMB2757 encodes a WD repeat protein required for embryo development in Arabidopsis. Plant Physiol 2005; 139(1):163-73.
44. Li D, Roberts R. WD-repeat proteins: structure characteristics, biological function and their involvement in human diseases. Cell Mol Life Sci 2001; 58:2085-97.
45. Benjafield AV, Jeyasingam CL, Nyholt DR et al. G-Protein ß3 subunit gene (GNB3) variant in causation of essential hypertension Hypertension 1998; 32:1094-97.
46. Handschug K, Sperling S, Yoon SJK et al. Triple A syndrome is caused by mutations in AAAS, a new WD-repeat protein gene. Hum Mol Genet 2001; 10(3):283-90.
47. Rietzler M, Bittner M, Kolanus W et al. The human WD repeat protein WAIT-1 specifically interacts with the cytoplasmic tails of beta 7-integrins. J Biol Chem 1998; 273(42):27459-66.
48. Halder T, Pawelec G, Kirkin AF et al. Isolation of novel HLA-DR restricted potential tumor-associated antigens from the melanoma cell line FM3. Cancer Res 1997; 57(15):3238-44.
49. Honore B, Baandrup U, Nielsen S et al. Endonuclein is a cell cycle regulated WD-repeat protein that is up-regulated in adenocarcinoma of the pancreas. Oncogene 2002; 21(7):1123-29.
50. Chernova OB, Hunyadi A, Malaj E et al. A novel member of the WD-repeat gene family, WDR11, maps to the 10q26 region and is disrupted by a chromosome translocation in human glioblastoma cells. Oncogene 2001; 20(38):5378-92.
51. Polakis P. Wnt signaling and cancer. Genes Dev 2000; 14(15):1837-51.
52. Parisi MA, Doherty D, Eckert ML et al. AHI1 mutations cause both retinal dystrophy and renal cystic disease in Joubert syndrome. J Med Genet 2006; 43(4):334-39.

CHAPTER 3

A Brief History of the Coronin Family

Eugenio L. de Hostos*

What I'd like to do in this chapter is to share with you my recollections from the earliest days of coronin research and then to provide an overview of the still-developing story of this fascinating family of proteins.

Oktoberfest Beats Falling-Ball Viscometry

In the fall of 1989 I arrived as a postdoc in Guenther Gerisch's department at the Max Planck Institute for Biochemistry in Munich to start a project on actin-binding proteins from *Dictyostelium discoideum*. Angelika Noegel (University of Cologne) and Michael Schleicher (University of Munich) had at the time their own subgroups in the Gerisch department that had done some beautiful work in this area.[1] Schleicher's approach had been to purify proteins that affected actin polymerization, primarily using falling-ball viscometry and pyrene-actin fluorimetry as assays. Noegel had led the molecular biology aspects of the projects, which involved the cloning of the genes and their inactivation by gene disruption followed by the analysis of the mutants.

When I arrived in the lab, however, I found some general frustration with the fact that some of the proteins that had been purified based on dramatic effects on in vitro actin polymerization (e.g. severin) were at least partially redundant in *Dictyostelium*.[1-4] Thus, the loss of the proteins did not have much of an effect on the cells and did not generate a phenotype that could shed some light on the biological function of the proteins.

Another thing I found out very quickly was that there were no unclaimed actin-binding proteins in the department that I could get to work on right away and that I'd have to decide quickly on a way of finding my own. I didn't have the temperament of a biochemist and I wasn't too keen on the Schleicher approach which might require spending much of my precious time in Munich (especially during Oktoberfest) timing little steel balls falling through tubes filled with F-actin. I wasn't too enthusiastic either about the Gerisch proposal to raise monoclonal antibodies against a crude detergent-extracted cytoskeletal fraction and to screen them for interesting cytoskeletal localization by immunofluorescence. I wasn't entirely against this "get antibodies first and ask questions later" approach and I certainly wanted to learn how to make monoclonal antibodies (for which the Gerisch group was well known), but I just thought that raising mAbs against crude cytoskeletal fraction was too much of a shot in the dark. I thought a more specific, cleaner cytoskeletal fraction would be better and after some digging in the literature I came across a cytoskeletal preparation called the "contracted pellet" that had been used previously[5] to purify a number of cytoskeletal proteins. This protocol involved the preparation of a highly concentrated cytoplasmic fraction from which acto-myosin could be precipitated, along with associated proteins.

My version of the preparation was similar to those described previously and consisted mostly of actin and myosin (heavy chain plus two light chains), a previously characterized 30 kD actin cross-linker[5] and two bands of 17 kD and 55 kD, respectively. Nothing was known about the latter two proteins but hoping that they would be cytoskeletal I carried on with their characterization. I

*Eugenio L. de Hostos—Molecular Imaging Program, Stanford University, School of Medicine. The James H. Clark Center E-150 318 Campus Drive, Stanford, CA 94305. Email: hostos@pacbell.net

The Coronin Family of Proteins, edited by Christoph S. Clemen, Ludwig Eichinger and Vasily Rybakin. ©2008 Landes Bioscience and Springer Science+Business Media.

purified the two proteins further from the contracted pellet fraction and right away used them to immunize mice and to get some peptide sequence. It was not long before we had plenty of hybridomas producing antibodies against the proteins and enough peptide sequence to suggest that the proteins were novel. The immunofluorescence images we obtained with the antibodies gave us the first indication that we had stumbled across something interesting. Anti-p55 gave stunning images of actin-rich structures in the cells including crown-shaped protrusions on the surface of the cells, for which I decided to name the protein (*corona* is Latin for crown). The antibodies against p17 gave an interesting but less glamorous labeling pattern, showing general enrichment throughout the cell cortex.[6] The 17 kD protein was named coactosin and is a member of the ADF/cofilin family with an interesting story of its own.[7]

We were all excited about the labeling pattern that anti-p55 gave but given all the previous work in the department on other cytoskeletal proteins that was based on a biochemical activity, there was some skepticism about this arriviste protein. Initially, I couldn't even show much binding to actin, the interaction being very sensitive to the concentration of NaCl. Fortunately, around that time I had a chance to talk to Ron Vale (University of California, San Francisco) on the long drive to a meeting in Austria. Vale, who had first characterized kinesins, suggested that I should try K-glutamate instead of NaCl, since K+ and glutamate were more representative of the intracellular milieu than were Na$^+$ and Cl$^-$. This did the trick and I was able to show binding of coronin to F-actin, but found no obvious effect on the polymerization of G-actin or an effect such as severing or cross-linking of F-actin. I think this finding was the source of some *Schadenfreude* among the falling-ball crowd in the department but I didn't know any better than to remain optimistic and, fortunately, molecular biology soon made the coronin story a lot more interesting.

Using the excellent mAbs that we had made I was able to quickly clone coronin cDNAs from an expression library. To my chagrin vis-à-vis the biochemists, it didn't look like any actin-binding protein that had been sequenced before. Intriguingly it had homology to, of all things, the β subunits of the trimeric G-proteins (Gβ). We found five repeats of the WD motif that was characteristic of the Gβ subunits, in which it was repeated seven times. This similarity was puzzling but full of intriguing possibilities. The homology to Gβ led to some wild speculation that perhaps coronin was a link between the actin cytoskeleton and the G protein-coupled cAMP receptor that triggered chemotaxis in *Dictyostelium*. Buoyed by these ideas, but in the absence of any biochemical evidence to support the hypothesis, we sent the manuscript describing the initial characterization of coronin to Nature, which, rightly so, rejected the paper for not being substantial enough.

A more subdued manuscript was eventually published[8] but for more substance I turned to molecular biology, with which I was most comfortable. With a cDNA in one hand and a recent paper[9] describing a new, faster and more efficient method for gene disruption in the other, I quickly set about the job of finding out what coronin did in the cell. The transfection worked like a charm and within a week the technician working with me reported some strange looking cells in our plates: monstrous cells several times the size of normal cells and containing many nuclei. Knocking genes out in *Dictyostelium* was then still something of an event and we were sitting on top of the world when we confirmed the gene disruption and the absence of coronin with our antibodies.

In our characterization of the mutant we focused on chemotaxis and cytokinesis.[10] Using image analysis software developed in the department we found that the mutants migrated and oriented properly in cAMP gradients but moved less effectively. I was more intrigued by the cytokinesis defect, manifested by a very photogenic phenotype. In studying this defect we found that unlike myosin II mutants, the coronin mutants were not as severely impaired in performing cytokinesis,[9,11] they just didn't seem to be able to do so as effectively as normal cells. Interestingly, the coronin mutants grew fairly well in liquid, while the myosin mutants lysed after a few rounds of mitosis without cytokinesis. We interpreted this to mean that while coronin might have a role in the cleavage furrow, part of the effect on cytokinesis was due to the role played in the process by cell locomotion (and hence daughter cell separation), which was clearly affected in the mutants.[10,12]

The defect in locomotion and cytokinesis left little doubt that coronin was playing an important role in the actin cytoskeleton but the phenotype did not give a clear indication of what coronin was doing. There was an intriguing subtlety to the phenotype, in that the cells were quite viable and seemed to be able to do everything wild-type cells could do, just not as quickly or effectively. Coronin appeared to play a non-essential but significant accessory role in a variety of actin-based processes. In addition, the presence of the WD repeats gave us a reason and, lacking a biochemical activity, an excuse to speculate that whatever coronin did to actin happened through the interaction with other proteins. Putting these ideas together, the best we could say for a long time and with a lot of hand waving, was that coronin was affecting "cytoskeletal reorganization" and "actin dynamics" in partnership with other proteins (Fig. 1A).[10]

Coronin Becomes a Real Protein

Despite the remarkable phenotype caused by the loss of coronin, the lack of a biochemical explanation or evidence for homologous proteins in other organisms resulted in coronin being regarded as just an intriguing curiosity from slime molds when I left Munich in 1992. Within a couple of years, however, work by a number of labs would start making it a bona fide member of the cytoskeletal world.

Markus Maniak (University of Kassel), who had earlier done his PhD under Wolfgang Nellen in the Gerisch department, returned to Munich and quickly made good use of a fabulous new tool known as green fluorescent protein (GFP) to tag coronin and follow its dynamic localization in vivo.[13,14] This was the first reported fusion of GFP to a component of the actin cytoskeleton and the beautiful movies provided insight into the role of coronin as well as demonstrating the huge potential of GFP for tracking dynamic processes in cells. The movies showed clearly the involvement of coronin with the actin network at the leading edge of migrating cells, in the cortical crowns and

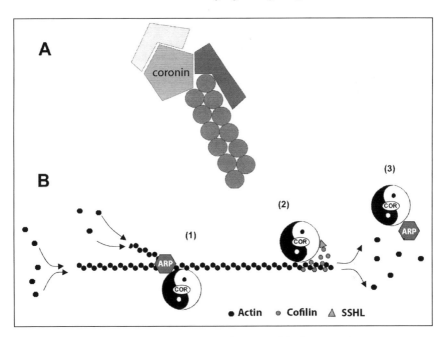

Figure 1. Models of coronin function. A) Speculative model of coronin function (1995, E. L. de Hostos, unpublished) suggesting the involvement of coronin in actin dynamics in partnership with other actin-binding proteins. B) Current model of core coronin functions.[17,38,39,41] 1) Coronin recruits Arp2/3 complex to existing actin filaments and promotes the formation of branches. 2) Coronin stimulates the activity of cofilin to depolymerize actin filaments at their pointed (ADP-actin containing ends) directly, or by recruiting the SSH1L phosphatase. 3) In the absence of F-actin, coronin inhibits the nucleation activity of Arp2/3.

with the actin coat that forms around phagocytic cups and which is likely to be a driving force in their formation. GFP-coronin showed that within minutes of their formation, phagosomes shed their coat containing actin and coronin and that coronin relocalizes to the cell cortex.

In parallel with the GFP-coronin studies, the Gerisch group made an intriguing observation about the coronin knockout mutants. They found that these cells had an abnormally broad cell cortex and more F-actin than wild-type cells.[14] Furthermore, they showed that treatment with the barbed-end capping agent cytochalasin A could restore the cortex to a more normal configuration. In light of these results they interpreted the cell architecture and sluggishness of coronin mutants in terms of a role for coronin in promoting the disassembly of actin filaments.

The publication of the Maniak's beautiful coronin-GFP results was followed by the identification of the first coronin homolog,[15] a 57 kD protein from human and bovine immune tissues (coronin 1A, also known as coronin 1 and p57). In their characterization the authors also recognized that coronin had a coiled-coiled domain at the C-terminus, a feature that we had missed in our description of the *Dictyostelium* coronin and which has turned out to be almost universal in the coronin family and essential for oligomerization and some of its key interactions.[16-20] Finding coronin in mammals had a large impact on how this protein was perceived and allowed it to start shedding its status as a *Dictyostelium* curiosity. As it turns out, the discovery of coronin 1A in immune cells was just the beginning of one of the most interesting coronin stories.

Like *Dictyostelium* coronin, coronin 1A was found to be involved in phagocytosis. The protein was found to copurify with components of the NADPH oxidase (phox) complex, which assembles on the surface of phagosomes to generate superoxide aimed at killing pathogens caught inside.[21] Much like in *Dictyostelium*, phagosomes in immune cells such as neutrophils have a transient coat containing actin and coronin. Work on the mechanism by which mycobacteria survive phagocytosis by macrophages has also led to coronin 1A. Jean Pieters (University of Basel Biozentrum) and coworkers discovered that unlike phagosomes with heat-killed mycobacteria, phagosomes with viable mycobacteria retained the coat of actin and coronin 1A (TACO).[22] We will discuss this in more detail in a section below.

Core Function

Within a couple of years of the discovery of coronin 1A, similar proteins had been found in a variety of model organisms and additional coronins had been identified in mammals, including two close relatives of coronin 1A, coronin 1B and coronin 1C (the three have also been referred to in the literature as coronins 1, 2 and 3, respectively).[23-27] The ubiquity of coronins and, for some at least, an evolutionarily conserved role in the medically relevant process of phagocytosis brought coronins into the mainstream but did not clarify their function.

Since the coronin-null mutants of *Dictyostelium* moved and divided inefficiently and lacked the characteristic F-actin-rich crowns on their surface, I initially envisioned coronin as being involved in somehow enhancing actin polymerization or stabilizing actin filaments. As mentioned earlier, however, Gerisch and coworkers later came to an opposite, more educated hypothesis, one with a role for coronin in promoting the disassembly of actin-filaments and "balancing the activities of proteins that nucleate actin polymerization".[14] Gerisch was on to something but biochemical evidence would have to wait until the discovery of Crn1p and the Arp2/3 complex.

Coronin from budding yeast, Crn1p, was initially identified by an in silico homology search[28] and in parallel purified, surprisingly, by microtubule affinity chromatography[29]. Microtubule binding not withstanding, Crn1 turned out to be true to its other coronin relatives and shown to be intimately involved with the actin cytoskeleton. Bruce Goode (Brandeis University), then a postdoc with Georjana Barnes and David Drubin at Berkeley, showed for the first time evidence for a biochemical function: the stimulation of polymerization of pure actin and the bundling of actin filaments (as well as the cross-linking of these actin bundles to microtubules).[29] These properties, however, have turned out to be only a short preview on the functions of coronins in regulating actin dynamics.

For many years the actin cytoskeleton had been understood mostly in terms of a rather limited set of components and functions: actin (G and F), capping proteins, cross-linkers, severing proteins and, of course, myosin. But that construction set gained a whole new dimension with the discovery and initial characterization of the Arp2/3 complex.[30-32] Nucleation is the rate-limiting step in actin polymerization and therefore the generation of nucleation sites is a key regulatory step in the assembly of actin networks. Until the discovery of the Arp2/3 complex, the severing of actin filaments by proteins such as cofilin was thought to be the primary mechanism for generating nucleation sites and stimulating polymerization. Arp2/3 is a complex of seven proteins that drives the rapid de novo assembly of F-actin, by nucleating daughter filaments from the side of existing filaments and forming a branching meshwork.[33,34] Intriguingly, it was found that preparations of Arp2/3 from human neutrophils contained sub-stoichiometric amounts of coronin 1A, in addition to the seven subunits of the complex.[35] The presence of coronin in preparations of the Arp2/3 complex suggested, finally, a partnership through which coronin might be affecting "actin dynamics".

Bruce Goode and coworkers started to reveal the nature of this partnership when they found that Crn1p bound Arp2/3 via its coiled-coil and recruited it to the sides of pre-existing F-actin filaments. In the absence of pre-existing filaments they found, however, that Crn1p inhibited the actin-nucleating activity of the complex. Therefore, they proposed that coronin inhibits Arp2/3-mediated polymerization in the cytoplasm, but promotes nucleation and branching at the cell cortex.[17]

The prevalence and importance of the coronin-Arp2/3 partnership has been validated further by a number of studies.[36-39] Working with coronin 1B, James Bear's group (University of North Carolina) has shown that phosphorylation by protein kinase C (PKC) of a widely conserved serine residue (S2) inhibits the interaction of coronin with Arp2/3.[37] S2 phosphorylation has also been shown to control Arp2/3 interaction in coronin 1A.[40] Bear's group found that cells expressing coronin 1B with a phosphomimetic aspartate substitution (S2D) were sluggish and displayed reduced ruffling, as might be expected from a knockout.[37] Indeed, Rat2 cells depleted of coronin 1B by shRNA expression showed a consistent phenotype.[39] A key finding in this study was that retrograde flow of actin filaments from the cell periphery was drastically reduced. While the details as to exactly how the coronin-Arp2/3 partnership works are still being worked out, this observation illustrates clearly that one of its key functions is to regulate filament turnover.

Polymerization and depolymerization are two sides of the same coin (or filament, in this case), so what about the role of coronin in filament disassembly? Goode and coworkers had shown that while the deletion of Crn1p caused no overt phenotypes, it did cause a more severe synthetic phenotype when combined with alleles of cofilin (*cof1-22*) and actin (*act1-159*), which were known to reduce actin filament turn-over and stabilize F-actin in vivo.[29] The synthetic phenotypes observed would make sense if coronin had a role in depolymerization and its loss made things worse for the cells by reducing filament turnover even further. This interpretation was supported by evidence suggesting that in vitro Crn1p in fact synergizes with cofilin to promote filament disassembly (M. Gandhi and B. Goode, personal communication). Results consistent with this observation have come from the study of actin dynamics in the comet tails generated by *Listeria*.

A study aimed at purifying factors that would stimulate the otherwise weak in vitro activity of cofilin to depolymerize the actin tails identified two proteins, coronin 1A and the actin-binding protein Aip1 that can do so, separately and in combination.[41] The authors suggested that coronin stimulates cofilin activity indirectly, by binding to actin filaments and altering their structure in a way that facilitates the binding of cofilin.[41] Work on coronin 1C[36] showing that antibodies directed against coronin will co-immunoprecipitate cofilin, however, has suggested a direct interaction with cofilin as well. More recent work from the Bear lab, however, found no evidence for enhanced binding of cofilin to F-actin in the presence of coronin 1A or 1B.[38] Instead they found that coronin binding actually protected the actin filaments from cofilin-induced depolymerization.[38] They have proposed that coronin 1B can enhance cofilin activity in vivo by directing the localization of the slingshot phosphatase (SSH1L) to lamellipodia, where it can activate cofilin by dephosphorylation.[39]

The picture of how coronins regulate actin filament turnover is complicated and not yet complete, but it is clear that it is involved at both ends, so to speak, in filament assembly and filament disassembly (Fig. 1B). I think that one of the surprises in the picture that is emerging is that F-actin itself is one of coronin's key partners. In other words, rather than being just a substrate, as it is for other actin-binding proteins, F-actin seems to be an active partner that regulates coronin function. Not only does it appear that coronin can sense the presence or absence of F-actin and regulate Arp2/3 accordingly,[17] there is evidence that coronin can also distinguish the nucleotide state of the F-actin involved. Bear's group has shown[38] that coronin 1B has much higher affinity for ATP-F-actin than for ADP-F-actin, an observation that implies that coronin can determine whether it is at the ATP-actin-containing barbed end of filaments or the ADP-actin-containing pointed end. It remains a major future challenge to put together a model that harmonizes all of the biochemical results with all of the phenotypic observations, but I think that we are starting to see a sophisticated coronin-based system for fine-tuning actin turnover in response to temporal and spatial cues. In Chapter III-1 Bruce Goode will delve into this topic further.

All in the Family

One recurring question about the coronin family is how conserved are the interactions of coronins with actin? Even though our knowledge of the family is far from comprehensive, I think that it is fair to say that interacting with actin is ancestral to the family and that actin-regulatory functions are likely to have evolved early and been retained by many members of the family.[16,26,42] That said, I think there is likely to be significant diversity in the details of their actin-regulatory functions, both in terms of inputs (i.e., signals and partners) and in terms of outputs (i.e., targets). This diversity may support the specialization of different coronins for a wide range of actin-based processes (e.g., cell migration vs phagocytosis) in different cell types or even in the economy of the same cell. Some coronins appear to have evolved out of their actin-regulatory functions completely but I suspect that if we look hard enough we will always find actin in their circle of protein partners. In considering coronin diversity, I like to visualize coronin functions in terms of a model like the structure of the earth, with ancestral functions at the core and accessory functions in layers more or less removed from the core functions (Fig. 2).

The coronin family shows its greatest diversity in mammals, in which it can be divided into three types.[16] Type I includes coronins 1A, 1B and 1C [and coronin 6; for latest knowledge on coronin phylogeny see chapter II-2], which like Crn1p from yeast, have been shown to be involved

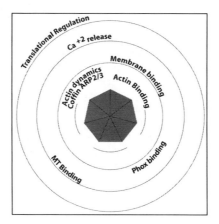

Figure 2. Range of coronin activities. The activities of the coronins range from the ancestral core functions mediated by actin binding and affecting actin turnover to accessory functions such as microtubule (MT) and membrane binding. Additional functions may include the regulation of Ca^{2+} release and even transcriptional regulation.

in the regulation of actin dynamics through Arp2/3 and cofilin (core functions) and thus belong in the same functional group. *Dictyostelium* coronin is almost certainly another member of this group, but this has not been proven biochemically.

Coronin 1A is expressed preferentially in immune tissues along with coronin 1B and 1C which are expressed ubiquitously.[16,26] With one possible exception, the reports describing the phenotype of cells in which these coronins have been eliminated or inhibited are similar and consistent with the phenotype of the original *Dictyostelium* knockout mutants. The thymocytes from knockout mice lacking coronin 1A are impaired in chemotaxis and locomotion in general[40] and, interestingly, they tend to undergo apoptosis in vivo. This apoptotic phenotype is thought to be a consequence of excess of F-actin disrupting mitochondrial integrity.[40,43] In human neutrophils, coronin 1A lacking the coiled-coil domain has a dominant-negative effect and disrupts phagocytosis, chemotaxis, spreading and adhesion.[19,20] Surprisingly, however, the truncated coronin has no effect on the secretion or the activation of the phox complex, with which coronin is thought to associate. Rat2 cells in which coronin 1B had been depleted by shRNA also show impaired motility.[38] Work on coronin 1C using dominant negative mutants and siRNA has shown results similar to those seen with coronins 1A and 1B, as well as an effect on cytokinesis.[36]

The one exception to this consistent spectrum of phenotypes comes from studies of another lineage of knockout mice lacking coronin 1A.[44] Surprisingly, the study concluded that coronin 1A was dispensable for actin-mediated processes such as motility. This is an intriguing observation but I suspect that it is an issue of penetrance rather than a fundamental discrepancy with the results obtained by other groups. More importantly, however, this study confirmed the hypothesis mentioned earlier that coronin 1A is required for mycobacteria to survive in the phagosomes of infected macrophages.[22] Initially it was speculated that the retention of actin and coronin around phagosomes might prevent the fusion with lysosomes, thus protecting the mycobacteria from destruction. Work with cells from the knockout mice has shown, however, that the role of coronin 1A in this process goes beyond the cytoskeletal realm. Retention of coronin 1A leads to the Ca^{2+}-dependent activation of calcineurin (protein phosphatase 3), which in turn prevents the fusion of lysosomes with the phagosome.[44] In the context of phagocytosis then coronin 1A seems to have acquired a slew of accessory functions beyond its core functions. These include actin-independent binding to the cholesterol-rich phagosome membrane (through the WD domain),[45] binding to the phox complex,[21] an undefined role in the release of Ca^2 required for calcineurin activation.[44] Jean Pieters will discuss this remarkable story in more detail in Chapter IV-1.

While the results concerning Type I coronins are painting a mostly consistent story about their role in actin dynamics, much less is know about those classified as Type II (coronin 2A and 2B) and Type III (coronin 7).[16] As we learn more about them they are likely to provide additional examples of functionality distant or completely divorced from the core functions. Coronin 2B (ClipinC) from brain has been shown to bind F-actin and the actin and membrane-binding protein vinculin, but it is not really known what role it plays in the neuronal cytoskeleton.[46] Coronin 2A may be up to something far removed from its ancestral functions and has been implicated in transcriptional regulation, due to its presence in the nuclear receptor corepressor (N-CoR).[47] A role in transcription may seem "way out there" in the outer reaches of coronin space, but curiously, the only protein detected (other than coronin itself) in a two-hybrid screen using full-length *Dictyostelium* coronin as a bait was a protein (DB10 or coronin binding protein; XP_643969) that showed a sharp nuclear localization when tagged with GFP (D. Benhayon, W. Gu and E. L. de Hostos unpublished).

Type III coronins are different from other coronins in that they consist of two coronins fused in tandem but lacking coiled-coiled domains. In humans, they are represented by coronin 7. Type III coronins from *Caenorhabditis* (POD-1)[48] and *Drosophila* (Dpod1)[49] have been shown to be involved with actin but seem participate in different processes. The embryonic-lethal phenotype of POD-1 mutants suggests that it is required for polarized membrane trafficking necessary for the establishment of anterior-posterior polarity in the embryo.[42,48] Consistent with this phenotype, coronin 7 is associated with the Golgi apparatus and has been implicated in vesicle trafficking[42,50,51] (see also chapter III-4 by Rybakin). So far coronin 7 has not been found to interact with actin but I am holding out for the possibility that future research will show it to be the exception that proves the rule that all coronins interact with actin.

Drosophila Dpod1 does not seem to participate in membrane trafficking like POD-1 but it can bind microtubules, a function that coronins seem to have acquired more than once. Crn1p and Dpod1 both have a microtubule-binding domain with homology to MAP1B that lets them crosslink microtubules to actin-filaments.[48,49]

Full of Surprises

WD repeats were, in a way, where the coronin story started and so I can't end this review without a word about the structure of coronins. The archetypal WD repeat proteins are the Gβ subunits, which have seven repeats and fold into a seven-bladed β-propeller.[52,53] Although motif searches only identify five canonical WD repeats in coronins, the crystal structure of coronin 1A has shown that there are two cryptic WD repeats and that like the Gβ subunits, the protein folds into a seven-bladed β-propeller structure.[54] So while coronin did not turn out to be a direct link between G-protein coupled receptors and the cytoskeleton, they have turned out to be more structurally similar to the Gβ subunits than was originally thought based on sequence homology.

The WD repeat domain has been shown to be involved in a number of important interactions: binding actin filaments[36,38] (although the coiled-coil can too),[17] phosphorylation by protein kinase C (PKC)[37] and actin-independent binding of membranes.[45] The perception of the WD repeat domain as a nexus of protein-protein interactions has not been substantiated, but that may still happen, as more interactions (e.g., Golgi, Ca^{2+} release, SSH1L) are mapped on the protein structure. It is clear, however, that even though the WD domain with its β-propeller structure wins the crystallographic beauty contest, the humble coiled-coil domain is not just a "structural" element and is responsible for some key interactions such as binding actin and the Arp2/3 complex.[17] Coronins are, indeed, full of surprises.

Looking back over 16 years of work on coronins, what strikes me the most is how close, yet how very far away we were in the beginning to understanding the function of this interesting family of proteins. From the time we first got a look at the *Dictyostelium* coronin sequence and saw the WD repeats we guessed that the protein was likely to interact and perform its function through multiple binding partners. Later, based on the phenotype of the *Dictyostelium* mutants, we went on guessing and suggested that coronin had something to do with actin dynamics. Yet it has taken years of intricate work and the discovery of new proteins to substantiate this and come to a fair understanding of how coronins perform their core functions.

For someone who planted a small seed years ago and has watched others cultivate it, it is satisfying to see how the coronin story has grown and different strands of evidence have started to come together so neatly. Most rewarding is the fact that coronin is turning out to be an important player in the key process of actin turnover. But not all is said and done and as in any good family saga, I think that this story has a long way to go and this quirky family will continue to reward researchers with unexpected results and new insights into fundamental cellular processes.

Acknowledgement

The author would like to thank Bruce Goode, Jim Bear and Angela Barth for helpful discussions, and Chris Franklin for help with Figure 2.

References

1. Gerisch G, Noegel AA, Schleicher M. Genetic alteration of proteins in actin-based motility systems. Annu Rev Physiol 1991; 53:607-28.
2. Andre E, Brink M, Gerisch G et al. A Dictyostelium mutant deficient in severin, an F-actin fragmenting protein, shows normal motility and chemotaxis. J Cell Biol 1989; 108:985-95.
3. Wallraff E, Schleicher M, Modersitzki M et al. Selection of Dictyostelium mutants defective in cytoskeletal proteins: use of an antibody that binds to the ends of alpha-actinin rods. EMBO J 1986; 5:61-7.

4. Brink M, Gerisch G, Isenberg G et al. A Dictyostelium mutant lacking an F-actin cross-linking protein, the 120-kD gelation factor. J Cell Biol 1990; 111:1477-89.
5. Fechheimer M, Taylor DL. Isolation and characterization of a 30,000-dalton calcium-sensitive actin cross-linking protein from Dictyostelium discoideum. J Biol Chem 1984; 259:4514-20.
6. de Hostos EL, Bradtke B, Lottspeich F et al. Coactosin, a 17 kDa F-actin binding protein from Dictyostelium discoideum. Cell Motil Cytoskeleton 1993; 26:181-91.
7. Rakonjac M, Fischer L, Provost P et al. Coactosin-like protein supports 5-lipoxygenase enzyme activity and up-regulates leukotriene A4 production. Proc Natl Acad Sci USA 2006; 103:13150-5.
8. de Hostos EL, Bradtke B, Lottspeich F et al. Coronin, an actin binding protein of Dictyostelium discoideum localized to cell surface projections, has sequence similarities to G protein beta subunits. EMBO J 1991; 10:4097-104.
9. Manstein DJ, Titus MA, De Lozanne A et al. Gene replacement in Dictyostelium: generation of myosin null mutants. EMBO J 1989; 8:923-32.
10. de Hostos EL, Rehfuess C, Bradtke B et al. Dictyostelium mutants lacking the cytoskeletal protein coronin are defective in cytokinesis and cell motility. J Cell Biol 1993; 120:163-73.
11. De Lozanne A, Spudich JA. Disruption of the Dictyostelium myosin heavy chain gene by homologous recombination. Science 1987; 236:1086-91.
12. Nagasaki A, de Hostos EL, Uyeda TQ. Genetic and morphological evidence for two parallel pathways of cell-cycle-coupled cytokinesis in Dictyostelium. J Cell Sci 2002; 115:2241-51.
13. Maniak M, Rauchenberger R, Albrecht R et al. Coronin involved in phagocytosis: dynamics of particle-induced relocalization visualized by a green fluorescent protein Tag. Cell 1995; 83:915-24.
14. Gerisch G, Albrecht R, Heizer C et al. Chemoattractant-controlled accumulation of coronin at the leading edge of Dictyostelium cells monitored using a green fluorescent protein-coronin fusion protein. Curr Biol 1995; 5:1280-5.
15. Suzuki K, Nishihata J, Arai Y et al. Molecular cloning of a novel actin-binding protein, p57, with a WD repeat and a leucine zipper motif. FEBS Lett 1995; 364:283-8.
16. Uetrecht AC, Bear JE. Coronins: the return of the crown. Trends Cell Biol 2006; 16:421-6.
17. Humphries CL, Balcer HI, D'Agostino JL et al. Direct regulation of Arp2/3 complex activity and function by the actin binding protein coronin. J Cell Biol 2002; 159:993-1004.
18. Asano S, Mishima M, Nishida E. Coronin forms a stable dimer through its C-terminal coiled coil region: an implicated role in its localization to cell periphery. Genes Cells 2001; 6:225-35.
19. Yan M, Collins RF, Grinstein S et al. Coronin-1 function is required for phagosome formation. Mol Biol Cell 2005; 16:3077-87.
20. Yan M, Di Ciano-Oliveira C, Grinstein S et al. Coronin function is required for chemotaxis and phagocytosis in human neutrophils. J Immunol 2007; 178:5769-78.
21. Grogan A, Reeves E, Keep N et al. Cytosolic phox proteins interact with and regulate the assembly of coronin in neutrophils. J Cell Sci 1997;110(Pt 24):3071-81.
22. Ferrari G, Langen H, Naito M et al. A coat protein on phagosomes involved in the intracellular survival of mycobacteria. Cell 1999; 97:435-47.
23. Zaphiropoulos PG, Toftgard R. cDNA cloning of a novel WD repeat protein mapping to the 9q22.3 chromosomal region. DNA Cell Biol 1996; 15:1049-56.
24. Terasaki AG, Ohnuma M, Mabuchi I. Identification of actin-binding proteins from sea urchin eggs by F-actin affinity column chromatography. J Biochem (Tokyo) 1997; 122:226-36.
25. Tardieux I, Liu X, Poupel O et al. A Plasmodium falciparum novel gene encoding a coronin-like protein which associates with actin filaments. FEBS Lett 1998; 441:251-6.
26. de Hostos EL. The coronin family of actin-associated proteins. Trends Cell Biol 1999; 9:345-50.
27. Okumura M, Kung C, Wong S et al. Definition of family of coronin-related proteins conserved between humans and mice: close genetic linkage between coronin-2 and CD45-associated protein. DNA Cell Biol 1998; 17:779-87.
28. Heil-Chapdelaine RA, Tran NK, Cooper JA. The role of Saccharomyces cerevisiae coronin in the actin and microtubule cytoskeletons. Curr Biol 1998; 8:1281-4.
29. Goode BL, Wong JJ, Butty AC et al. Coronin promotes the rapid assembly and cross-linking of actin filaments and may link the actin and microtubule cytoskeletons in yeast. J Cell Biol 1999; 144:83-98.
30. Mullins RD, Stafford WF, Pollard TD. Structure, subunit topology and actin-binding activity of the Arp2/3 complex from Acanthamoeba. J Cell Biol 1997; 136:331-43.
31. Welch MD, Iwamatsu A, Mitchison TJ. Actin polymerization is induced by Arp2/3 protein complex at the surface of Listeria monocytogenes. Nature 1997; 385:265-9.
32. Machesky LM, Atkinson SJ, Ampe C et al. Purification of a cortical complex containing two unconventional actins from Acanthamoeba by affinity chromatography on profilin-agarose. J Cell Biol 1994; 127:107-15.
33. Mullins RD, Pollard TD. Structure and function of the Arp2/3 complex. Curr Opin Struct Biol 1999; 9:244-9.

34. Pollard TD, Borisy GG. Cellular motility driven by assembly and disassembly of actin filaments. Cell 2003; 112:453-65.
35. Machesky LM, Reeves E, Wientjes F et al. Mammalian actin-related protein 2/3 complex localizes to regions of lamellipodial protrusion and is composed of evolutionarily conserved proteins. Biochem J 1997; 328(Pt 1):105-12.
36. Rosentreter A, Hofmann A, Xavier CP et al. Coronin 3 involvement in F-actin-dependent processes at the cell cortex. Exp Cell Res 2007; 313:878-95.
37. Cai L, Holoweckyj N, Schaller MD et al. Phosphorylation of coronin 1B by protein kinase C regulates interaction with Arp2/3 and cell motility. J Biol Chem 2005; 280:31913-23.
38. Cai L, Makhov AM, Bear JE. F-actin binding is essential for coronin 1B function in vivo. J Cell Sci 2007; 120:1779-90.
39. Cai L, Marshall TW, Uetrecht AC et al. Coronin 1B coordinates Arp2/3 complex and cofilin activities at the leading edge. Cell 2007; 128:915-29.
40. Foger N, Rangell L, Danilenko DM et al. Requirement for coronin 1 in T-lymphocyte trafficking and cellular homeostasis. Science 2006; 313:839-42.
41. Brieher WM, Kueh HY, Ballif BA et al. Rapid actin monomer-insensitive depolymerization of Listeria actin comet tails by cofilin, coronin and Aip1. J Cell Biol 2006; 175:315-24.
42. Rybakin V, Clemen CS. Coronin proteins as multifunctional regulators of the cytoskeleton and membrane trafficking. Bioessays 2005; 27:625-32.
43. Dustin ML. Immunology. When F-actin becomes too much of a good thing. Science 2006; 313:767-8.
44. Jayachandran R, Sundaramurthy V, Combaluzier B et al. Survival of mycobacteria in macrophages is mediated by coronin 1-dependent activation of calcineurin. Cell 2007; 130:37-50.
45. Gatfield J, Albrecht I, Zanolari B et al. Association of the leukocyte plasma membrane with the actin cytoskeleton through coiled coil-mediated trimeric coronin 1 molecules. Mol Biol Cell 2005; 16:2786-98.
46. Nakamura T, Takeuchi K, Muraoka S et al. A neurally enriched coronin-like protein, ClipinC, is a novel candidate for an actin cytoskeleton-cortical membrane-linking protein. J Biol Chem 1999; 274:13322-7.
47. Yoon HG, Chan DW, Huang ZQ et al. Purification and functional characterization of the human N-CoR complex: the roles of HDAC3, TBL1 and TBLR1. EMBO J 2003; 22:1336-46.
48. Rappleye CA, Paredez AR, Smith CW et al. The coronin-like protein POD-1 is required for anterior-posterior axis formation and cellular architecture in the nematode caenorhabditis elegans. Genes Dev 1999; 13:2838-51.
49. Rothenberg ME, Rogers SL, Vale RD et al. Drosophila pod-1 crosslinks both actin and microtubules and controls the targeting of axons. Neuron 2003; 39:779-91.
50. Rybakin V, Stumpf M, Schulze A et al. Coronin 7, the mammalian POD-1 homologue, localizes to the Golgi apparatus. FEBS Lett 2004; 573:161-7.
51. Rybakin V, Gounko NV, Spate K et al. Crn7 interacts with AP-1 and is required for the maintenance of Golgi morphology and protein export from the Golgi. J Biol Chem 2006; 281:31070-8.
52. Lambright DG, Sondek J, Bohm A et al. The 2.0 A crystal structure of a heterotrimeric G protein. Nature 1996; 379:311-9.
53. Wall MA, Coleman DE, Lee E et al. The structure of the G protein heterotrimer Gi alpha 1 beta 1 gamma 2. Cell 1995; 83:1047-58.
54. Appleton BA, Wu P, Wiesmann C. The crystal structure of murine coronin-1: a regulator of actin cytoskeletal dynamics in lymphocytes. Structure 2006; 14:87-96.

CHAPTER 4

Molecular Phylogeny and Evolution of the Coronin Gene Family

Reginald O. Morgan* and M. Pilar Fernandez

Abstract

The coronin gene family comprises seven vertebrate paralogs and at least five unclassified subfamilies in nonvertebrate metazoa, fungi and protozoa, but no representatives in plants or distant protists. All known members exhibit elevated structural conservation in two unique domains of unknown function (DUF1899 and DUF1900) interspaced by three canonical WD40 domains (plus additional pseudo domains) that form part of a 7-bladed β-propeller scaffold, plus a C-terminal variable "coiled coil domain" responsible for oligomerization. Phylogenetic analysis of the N-terminal conserved region in known members (i.e. 420 aa in 250 taxa) established the origin of the founding monomeric unit and a dimeric paralog in unicellular eukaryotes. The monomeric ancestor duplicated to two distinct lineages in basal metazoa and later propagated during the whole genome duplications in primitive chordates 450-550 million years ago to form six vertebrate-specific genes. The delineation of 12 subfamily clades in distinct phyla provided a rational basis for proposing a simplified, universal nomenclature for the coronin family in accordance with evolutionary history, structural relationships and functional divergence.

Comparative genomic analysis of coronin subfamily locus maps and gene organization provided corroboratory evidence for their chromosomal dispersal and structural relatedness. Statistical analysis of evolutionary sequence conservation by profile hidden Markov models (pHMM) and the prediction of Specificity Determining Positions (SDPpred) helped to characterize coronin domains by highlighting structurally conserved sites relevant to coronin function and subfamily divergence. The incorporation of such evolutionary information into 3D models facilitated the distinction between candidate sites with a structural role versus those implicated in dynamic, actin-related cytoskeletal interactions. A highly conserved "KGD" motif identified in the coronin DUF1900 domain has been observed in other actin-binding proteins such as annexins and is a potential ligand for integrins and C2 domains known to be associated with structural and signalling roles in the membrane cytoskeleton. Molecular evolution studies provide a comprehensive overview of the structural history of the coronin gene family and a systematic methodology to gain deeper insight into the function(s) of individual members.

Introduction

Biological and molecular sequence data describing the coronin gene family provide intriguing but limited information about their species distribution, expression profiles and structural features relevant to function.[1-3] A comprehensive phylogenetic analysis can be instructive to document gene family history, rationalize its nomenclature and fully appreciate the diversity and relatedness of individual members. Phylogenetic tree reconstruction is most reliable when supported by a broad

*Corresponding Author: Reginald O. Morgan—Department of Biochemistry and Molecular Biology, University of Oviedo and Instituto Universitario de Biotecnología de Asturias (IUBA), Oviedo, Spain E-33006. Email: morganreginald@uniovi.es

The Coronin Family of Proteins, edited by Christoph S. Clemen, Ludwig Eichinger and Vasily Rybakin. ©2008 Landes Bioscience and Springer Science+Business Media.

representation of authenticated homologs from completed genomes to ensure the identification of all paralogous genes and their cognate orthologs in different species. Computational rigor can be achieved by sequence analysis using various models of molecular evolution that generate maximum likelihood or bootstrap confidence values for the branching topology in which branch order and lengths are consistent with current knowledge about species evolution.

The focus on gene family evolution is of central importance to understanding gene and protein function because it assembles much relevant information from comparative genomics and proteomics. It yields statistically verifiable results for associating patterns and processes of structural change with functional determination and adaptation in the natural selection of species. In particular, the ability to define structure-function relationships among orthologous groups at the level of individual gene subfamilies is vital for comprehending the functional diversity and specificity of biological interactions for all members within a gene family. A multitude of algorithms in computational biology afford comprehensive, detailed views of genomic and proteomic data whilst others extend to comparative and investigative analyses. These can provide original insight into the structural features important for gene function because the targets of functional constraint can be deciphered from the statistics of evolutionary conservation and divergence. The elaboration of profile hidden Markov models (pHMM) and 3D structures that incorporate this information can be of predictive value and help to conceptualize and validate structure-function hypotheses worthy of empirical testing.

The vast quantity of molecular data being made available by ongoing genome sequencing projects provides a valuable resource that can be transformed, through computational biology techniques, into a knowledgebase relating evolutionary information to structure and function. The primary aims of the present study are to reconstruct the evolutionary relationships among all coronin subfamilies and use this as a framework to define their structural profiles with models that highlight functional relevance. Similar approaches can be contemplated for future studies to examine the molecular basis of coronin gene regulation or to evaluate coronin molecular interactions and conformational changes using in silico docking models.

Homolog Search and Assembly

Annotated protein databases such as UniProt (http://www.ebi.ac.uk/uniprot/) and PFAM (http://www.sanger.ac.uk/Software/Pfam/) and major sequence repositories such as National Center for Biotechnology Information (http://www.ncbi.nlm.nih.gov/), Ensembl (http://www.ensembl.org) and KEGG (http://www.genome.ad.jp/kegg/) provide direct access to many known, full-length coronin sequences. Additional sequences were retrieved using bioinformatic search tools such as BLAST, specialized databases such as Homologene (http://www.ncbi.nlm.nih.gov/sites/entrez?db=homologene) and other resources to search, assemble and cross-compare novel sequences from expressed transcripts (dbEST) and whole genome shotgun (WGS) traces. Organism specialized sequence databases from the Joint Genome Institute (http://www.jgi.doe.gov/), the Broad Institute (http://www.broad.mit.edu) and Washington University (http://genome.wustl.edu/) were accessed to reconstruct coronins of special interest for evolutionary placement. These included preliminary sequence assemblies of *Trichoplax adherens* (placozoa), *Monosiga brevicollis* (choanoflagellate), *Nematostella vectensis* (sea anemone), *Strongylocentrotus purpuratus* (purple urchin), *Branchiostoma floridae* (amphioxus), *Petromyzon marinus* (sea lamprey) and *Callorhincus milii* (elephant shark). Completed genome assemblies of key model vertebrates such as *Danio rerio* (zebrafish), *Xenopus tropicalis* (western clawed frog), *Gallus gallus* (chicken) and mammals such as platypus, shrew, bat, mouse, rat, cow, dog and various primates were also searched for annotated or predicted homologs. PSI-BLAST and HMMER search tools were used to confirm the absence of coronin domains in *Giardia intestinalis* and the plant kingdom.[4]

Approximately 250 full-length protein sequences spanning all major phyla were assembled into a multiple sequence alignment using the ClustalW utility in Molecular Evolutionary Genetics Analysis (MEGA) software version 4.0.[5] Phylogenetic tree construction was initially performed by MEGA4 neighbor-joining analysis of maximum likelihood distances for 5000 bootstrap alignments of 400 conserved sites (i.e., excluding the coiled coil region) in approximately 250 coronin proteins from a broad range of species. These results were validated by Bayesian analysis using Mr Bayes[6] and finally by maximum likelihood (ML) analysis using IQPNNI[7] v3.2 to yield the robust family trees for animal coronins (Fig. 1A) and those in unicellular eukaryotes (Fig. 1B).

Phylogenetic Analysis

The most recent diverging clades of monomeric coronins comprise six "vertebrate" subfamilies with species orthologs ranging from primitive fishes such as jawless Agnatha (e.g., sea lamprey), cartilaginous Chondrichthyes (e.g., elephant shark) and teleosts (e.g., zebrafish) to mammals, including human (Fig. 1A). They are designated here in reverse phylogenetic order as new coronins 1 through 6 (see nomenclature proposal section below) accompanied by their currently official nomenclature symbols CORO1B, 1C, 6, 1A, 2A and 2B. The common ancestry and species distribution of these subfamilies point to their probable divergence during the two postulated whole genome duplications (WGD) in primitive chordate ancestors. Duplicate coronin genes frequently observed in teleosts are a consequence of the extra tetraploidization event early in this lineage approximately 300-350 million years ago (Mya); examples shown include *Tetraodon nigroviridis* (green spotted pufferfish) coronin 2, *Gasterosteus aculeatus* (stickleback) and *Oryzias latipes* (Japanese medaka fish) coronin 3 and *Danio rerio* (zebrafish) coronin 6. The recently discovered coronin 3 (CORO6) gene is phylogenetically close to coronin 4 (CORO1A) but also shares some aspects of gene organization with the coronin 5 (CORO2A) ancestor (see later). It is pertinent to note that subfamily orthologs branch in the expected speciation order, except for occasional displacements due to the inclusion of some partial sequences. The branch lengths from bifurcation nodes together with the observed species distribution for each subfamily permit an estimation of the age and timing of these gene duplication and speciation events based on the horizontal time scale, which is quasi-linear due to rate variations in individual gene evolution. The formation of these expanded clades occurred in rapid succession around the time of emergence of the first vertebrate about 550 Mya, represented by the sea lamprey *Petromyzon marinus*. The earliest metazoan coronin monomers originated in two distinct clades of newly assigned invertebrate subfamilies 8 and 9 further to the left on the horizontal scale (Fig. 1A). These are represented at their basal position by the only two coronins detected in the 50 Mb genome assembly of *Trichoplax adherens*, a placozoan considered to represent the most primitive animal cell. Other invertebrates such as the Cnidarian *Nematostella vectensis*, the echinoderm *Strongylocentrotus purpuratus*, the cephalochordate *Branchiostoma floridae* and various insects all similarly possess two monomeric coronins within these two founding clades. The branching order shown in Figure 1A clarifies that invertebrate coronin 9 probably shared its most recent common ancestor with vertebrate coronins 5 and 6 (CORO2A and 2B), whilst a distinct common ancestor of invertebrate coronin 8 probably gave rise to vertebrate coronins 1-4.

The N- and C-terminal halves of all coronin 7 dimer representatives were aligned as separate taxa, beginning with their respective DUF1899 "domains of unknown function". They grouped into two adjacent clades rooted in the amoebae and fungal monomeric coronins (Fig. 1B), confirming that they originated from tandem duplication and fusion in a distant common ancestor, as opposed to the heterologous fusion of distinct monomers. The broad species distribution among protists, fungi and metazoa confirmed that this ubiquitous dimeric subfamily originated very early in coronin phylogeny and presumably conserves some basic cellular role. The relatively long branch lengths of some coronin 7 representatives reflect more extensive adaptive evolution (on horizontal scale) since the divergence from monomeric coronins. The basal branches in the coronin tree comprised monomeric coronins from fungi and diverse protozoa, the common ancestor of which formed coronin 7 via tandem duplication. Both maximum likelihood and independent bootstrap values at the bifurcation nodes of duplication or speciation gave generally strong support for the branching order. Minor variations in branch swapping were observed among basal taxa with low NJ-bootstrap support, such as the *Dictyostelium* representatives, but three well-defined clades distinguished the coronins from Alveolata, Fungi and Euglenozoa, which were assigned to

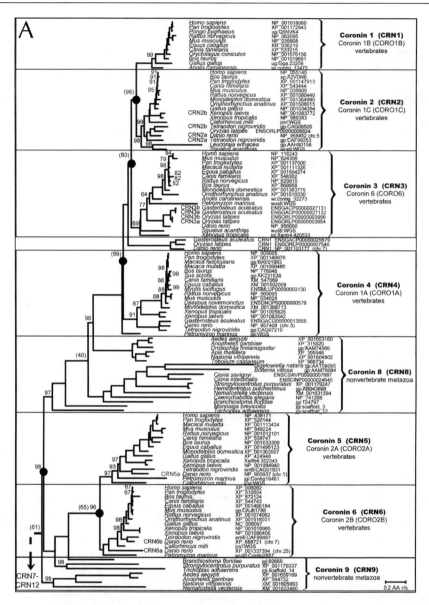

Figure 1. Phylogenetic tree of the coronin protein family. The input data consisted of an alignment comprising 420 aa in the common, conserved N-terminal region (i.e., DUF1899, WD40 and DUF1900 domains, excluding the coiled coil) from 250 species spanning the full diversity of known coronin structures. All sequences were obtained or derived from public databases and included some partial sequences from fish. Preliminary computation by the neighbor-joining algorithm of MEGA4 used pairwise maximum likelihood distances for 5000 bootstrapped alignments to approximate the given topology and branching confidence values shown as bootstrap percentages enclosed in brackets. The data were ultimately recomputed by the maximum likelihood program IQPNNI 3.2 with a gamma rate variation model to generate the displayed tree (split into two parts, A and B) with ML values of 100 at all unmarked nodes and actual ML values if less than 100. Legend continued on following page.

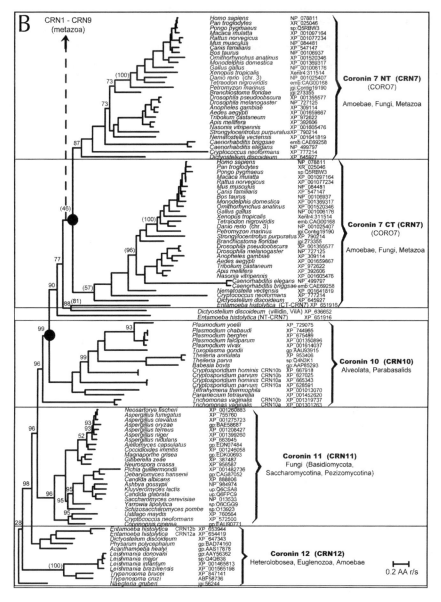

Figure 1, continued from previous page. Protein names and symbols correspond to the proposed new nomenclature (see text) followed by the current, official nomenclature (HGNC), using a and b suffixes to denote the products of duplicated genes in teleosts and *Xenopus laevis*. A) Vertebrate coronin subfamilies 1-6 diverged around the time of emergence of the first vertebrates, based on the observed species distribution and horizontal bifurcation points. Two novel and distinct clades for coronins 8 and 9 represented by nonvertebrate animals derived from a monomeric common ancestor prior to the emergence of the placozoan *Trichoplax adherens*. Gene duplication events are marked by solid circles at bifurcation nodes. B) Coronin 7 originated by tandem duplication and fusion of a protozoan monomeric coronin and exhibited the broadest species ubiquity. Monomeric coronins from Alveolata, Fungi and Euglenozoa formed three distinct subfamily clades at the base of the tree, which was rooted in the single coronin from the amoeboflagellate *Naegleria gruberi*.

new subfamilies 10, 11 and 12, respectively. The tree was rooted in the single coronin detected in *Naegleria gruberi*, a basal lineage of amoebae that transforms through a unique three-stage life cycle as amoeba, flagellate (with microtubule cytoskeleton) and cyst. Isolated cases of duplicate monomeric coronins in *Entamoeba*, *Cryptosporidium* and *Trichomonas* all appear to be relatively recent lineage-specific duplications. A unique duplicative fusion event in a common ancestor of *Dictyostelium* and *Entamoeba* gave rise to a novel gene fusion product of coronin with villin to form villidin (VilA, e.g., GenBank accession XP_636652) which is phylogenetically close to the coronin 7 C-terminal and coronin 10 Alveolata clades.

Nomenclature Proposal for the Coronin Gene Family

A successful nomenclature scheme for gene families is a priority objective of fundamental importance for the annotation and information exchange of emerging genomes. Ideally, it should be based on a comprehensive overview of each family and incorporate ample information about gene relationships in a clear, intuitive manner (Table 1). Original nomenclature compilations unified diverse terminologies derived from independent discoveries under the common name of coronins 1 through 5 assigned by a simple numbering scheme.[3] The currently official system from the Human Gene Nomenclature Committee (HGNC, http://www.genenames.org/) established the important precedent of an abbreviated gene symbol (CORO) as the primary unique identifier for information management and retrieval by electronic databases and attempted to define known gene relationships with enumeration by number-letter combinations (i.e., CORO1A, 1B, 1C, 2A, 2B, 6, 7). The apparent failure of the latter to be generally adopted stems from its intention of imparting more information by invoking awkward designations and by doing so prematurely such that later discovered coronins 6 and 7 appear dissociated and mislabeled. The lack of a broader overview of the family also precluded both systems from formally classifying many known invertebrate and protozoan coronins into a universal, systematic gene family nomenclature able to convey context, order and diversity.

The reconstruction of an ostensibly complete and properly rooted phylogenetic tree provides all the necessary information to devise a rational and universal nomenclature scheme that respects the principles and standards of systematic nomenclature and satisfies user needs for a simple, intuitive and informative system (Table 1). The delineation of major paralogous gene duplications and orthologous speciation events now makes it practicable to incorporate key evolutionary relationships as the scientific basis for associating structure with function, while preserving flexibility for future growth upon discovery of novel gene duplications or clade divisions. In order to maintain the gene name "coronin" with its changing usage and aliases during nomenclature development, a new symbol (e.g., "CRN") is needed to supplant the present symbol (CORO) and assume a dominant role for the immediate implementation and reliable dissemination of changes emanating from the HGNC via electronic database crosslinks to the worldwide research community. Its simple, strict format with contiguous number suffixes but without punctuation (i.e., no hyphens, spaces, periods, etc.) supplements other constant identifiers such sequence accessions, gene IDs or citation references to provide instant, unambiguous gene identification for all past and future scientific records, allowing the corresponding gene name to take a subordinate descriptive role. Lineage-specific gene duplicates would be designated with a standardized letter suffix (e.g., stickleback CRN3a and CRN3b) and alternative DNA transcripts can also be specified (e.g., human CRN2v1, CRN2v2, CRN2v3).

It is prudent to bear in mind that a universal nomenclature scheme with an intuitively logical scientific basis offers the greatest assurance for easy learning by newcomers to the field, faithful adherence by established investigators and an effective, enduring knowledgebase for biomedical research. The proposed nomenclature revision has attempted to combine the simple elegance of the original scheme with the identification power of a unique gene symbol and to build on these features by embracing the entire family and inculcating rational order so as to place all relevant genetic information in proper context. Any additional refinements to the proposed scheme should resist the tendency to grasp familiar relics, especially the deficiencies of outdated systems for reasons

Table 1. Nomenclature proposal for the coronin gene family, based on phylogenetic relationships[a]

Proposed New[b] Symbol, Name	Current Official[c] Symbol, Name	Prev. Alternate[d] Name Only	Other Alias Symbols; Names	Species Distribution (human locus map)
CRN1, coronin 1	CORO1B, coronin 1B	coronin 2	coronin se	Vertebrates (Hsa 11q13.1)
CRN2, coronin 2	CORO1C, coronin 1C	coronin 3	HCRNN4	Vertebrates (Hsa 12q24.1)
CRN3, coronin 3	CORO6, coronin 6	—	FLJ1487	Vertebrates (Hsa 17q11.2)
CRN4, coronin 4	CORO1A, coronin 1A	coronin 1	p57, TACO, ClipinA	Vertebrates (Hsa 16p11.2)
CRN5, coronin 5	CORO2A, coronin 2A	coronin 4	IR10, ClipinB, WDR2	Vertebrates (Hsa 9q22.3)
CRN6, coronin 6	CORO2B, coronin 2B	coronin 5	ClipinC	Vertebrates (Hsa 15q23)
CRN7, coronin 7	CORO7, coronin 7	—	P70, POD-1	Metazoa, Fungi, Amoebae (Hsa 16p13.3)
CRN8, coronin 8	—	—	—	Invertebrates, placozoa
CRN9, coronin 9	—	—	—	Invertebrates, placozoa
CRN10, coronin 10	—	—	—	Alveolata, Parabasalids
CRN11, coronin 11	—	—	Crn1p	Fungi (yeasts)
CRN12, coronin 12	—	—	—	Heterolobosea, Euglenzoa, Amoebae

[a]See phylogenetic analysis, Figs. 1A,B.
[b]Symbol designations have been sanctioned by the Human Gene Nomenclature Committee, but their usage has not yet been authorized as of this writing; see nomenclature discussion section.
[c]See HGNC website (http://www.genenames.org/) and ref. 1.
[d]From ref. 3.

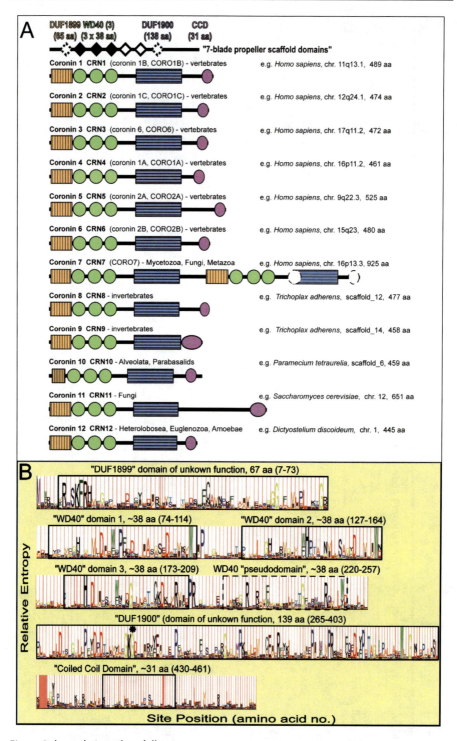

Figure 2, legend viewed on following page.

Figure 2, viewed on previous page. A) The domain organization of typical coronin proteins from 11 monomeric subfamilies and the dimeric coronin 7 are drawn to scale as sequential modules with the given names and lengths at the top. The characteristic structural domains include DUF1899, three WD40 domains as defined by the PFAM HMM model, a DUF1900 domain and a C-terminal coiled coil domain. Two additional "pseudo WD40" domains are indicated in the top schematic by open diamonds positioned after the true WD40 domains (the final one integrated within the DUF1900 domain) and dashed-line boxes localize two atypical domains flanking the WD40 repeats that collectively contribute to the 7-bladed β-propeller scaffold structure. Open symbols in the coronin 7 C-terminus refer to vestigial (i.e., eroded)/ WD40 and coiled coil domains. Proposed subfamily designations are accompanied by official symbols, species distribution and representative examples. B) The full-length coronin sequence logo was obtained from a profile hidden Markov model (pHMM) statistical representation of the amino acid distribution at each site in an alignment of the seven human coronins including coronin 7 N- and C-terminal halves aligned separately. Each column displays the expected amino acid distribution at that site and the total column height (entropy) reflects the level of functional constraint or information content at that site. The recognized domains are boxed separately and their sites of probable functional relevance can be inferred from the most prominent residue positions, such as the DUF1900 KGD motif (asterisk).

of nostalgia or personal convenience as this would surely defeat the long-term objective of attaining a coherent nomenclature system that consolidates ongoing research. The current official records and future changes in coronin nomenclature can always be consulted at the websites of the Human Gene Nomenclature Committee (http://www.genenames.org/) and Mouse Genome Informatics (http://www.informatics.jax.org/). This chapter utilizes the proposed new nomenclature (Table 1) based on original data (Figs. 1A,B) and accompanied by these official symbols.

Domain Structures and Hidden Markov Models

The primary structure characterization of coronin homologs was a prerequisite for validating homolog authenticity in the input alignment for phylogenetic analysis. We observed that coronin protein sequences aligned well with many highly conserved sites and few insertions and deletions, at least up to the C-terminal coiled coil region. All were confirmed to have congruent domain organization with two unique "Domains of Unknown Function" designated DUF1899 and DUF1900 (PFAM entries PF08953 and PF08954, respectively), separated by three canonical WD40 domains (i.e., defined by significant match scores to the PFAM-HMM model) and terminating in a coiled coil region of variable composition and length (Fig. 2A). The DUF1899 and DUF1900 coronin domains served as effective "bait" for the detection of distant coronin homologs and their unique, highly conserved structures likely play key roles in regulating actin dynamics in the cytoskeleton. The 3 canonical WD40, two "pseudo WD40" (i.e., vestigial, eroded domains) and two flanking "atypical domains" form the characteristic 7-bladed propeller scaffold structure of coronins.[8] One effective way to visualize the primary structure conservation or "molecular fingerprint" of these and other coronin domains is to use a multiple sequence alignment to generate a statistical "profile hidden Markov model" (pHMM) and transform it into a sequence logo (Fig. 2B). This composite logo outlines the amino acid distribution and over all conservation level at each site in a "typical" human coronin, based on the contribution of amino acids from all 8 human coronin monomers, including the component halves of coronin 7 separately in the alignment. Since the computation by HMMER[9] and LogoMat[10] also measures the relative probability that such a distribution of amino acid replacements would be found at random in nature, the total column height gives a measure of the entropy or information content that can be used to infer the functional importance of each site.

The 65-aa DUF1899 exhibits a prominent cluster of highly conserved (basic) amino acids at the amino terminus representing a coronin signature[1] that has been previously suggested to harbor a putative actin binding site just downstream of a phosphoserine modification site.[11,12] The three "true" WD40 domains that follow may vary in some coronin isoforms due to alternative exon splicing and two sequential "pseudo domains" exhibit much lower detectability by sequence

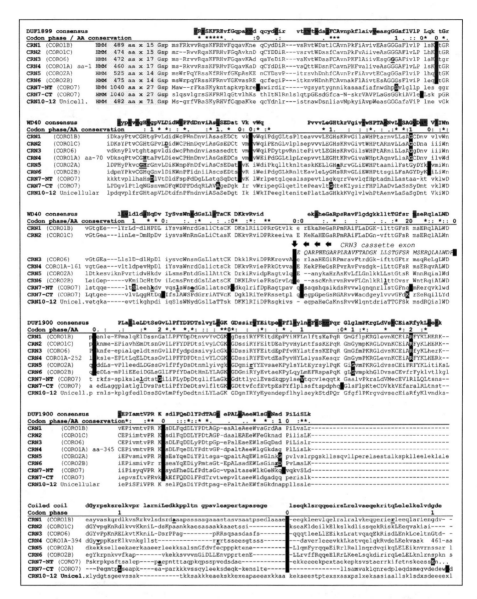

Figure 3. Multiple protein sequence alignment of consensus sequences for the major coronin subfamilies. Alignments of genus-species (Gsp) ortholog groups determined by phylogenetic analysis were used to generate hidden Markov models and a consensus protein sequence for each subfamily group, summarized beside the top set of names using new and official nomenclature. Capital letters denote greater than 50% conservation of the indicated amino acid, lower-case letters less than 50%. Sequence consensus models for the individual domains are shown above, with back-shaded amino acids denoting sites of subfamily divergence. Exon splice sites are indicated by rectangles and in reverse highlight of the encoded amino acid for the individual subfamilies (except for the protist-fungi group) with codon phase numbers (0, 1, 2) above those sites. Legend continued on following page.

Figure 3, continued from previous page. A cassette exon insertion site for an extra WD40 domain we observed in chicken and human expressed sequence tags of CRN3 isoforms is shown in the inset. Potential amino acid changes due to nonsynonymous nucleotide polymorphisms detected in humans are denoted by shaded, underlined amino acids. Putative isoforms reported for CRN2/CORO1C (N-terminal extensions) and CRN5/CORO2A (5'-untranslated region) are not included in the alignment and our sequence comparisons of transcript and genomic data indicated that their frequency of occurrence approached that of possible artefacts from EST library preparation.

search algorithms. While the typical WD40 domain (PFAM accession PF00400.23) generally has a conserved Gly-His early in the domain, internal and C-terminal Trp and several conserved Asp and Arg residues, other WD-like motifs in the center of DUF1899, a WL pair at the end of DUF1900 and atypical flanking domains may serve an analogous structural role together with the authentic WD40 domains.[8,13] This cluster is followed by a 139-aa DUF1900 domain unique to coronins, with well-defined conservation of Pro residues (inducing structural turns), charged Asp and Arg residues (disposed to external interactions) and a bulky aromatic Trp near its C-terminus. Our attention was drawn to the presence of a highly conserved "KGD" motif spanning an exon splice site in phase 1 of the codon (i.e., between the first and second nucleotide) that is constant in all coronins. This feature is identical to that observed in actin-binding members of the annexin gene family and identifies a potential ligand for interaction with membrane-bound integrins and signalling complexes enriched with C2-domain containing enzymes.[14] The C-terminal coiled coil region is most variable in composition and length, with additional insertions in coronin 5 and coronin 7 linker region and heterologous domain extensions (e.g., pleckstrin homology, gelsolin) in some yeast and amoeba monomeric coronins. The unique villidins of *Dictyostelium* (XP_636652) and *Entamoeba* (AF118397) are fascinating evolutionary anomalies resulting from gene fusion between the coronin and villin families of actin-binding proteins.

Structural Features of Coronin Subfamilies

The ability to decipher functionally relevant conserved sites or regions in the primary structure of the coronin family HMM (Fig. 2) can be obscured by subfamily divergence, so it is important to extend such analysis to ortholog groups of individual subfamilies to obtain distinctive molecular fingerprints for each. We therefore compiled pHMM models from multiple sequence alignments for each of the known subfamilies, including the invertebrate, fungal and protist monomeric coronins, to statistically validate new member classification and to conduct pairwise HMM-HMM comparisons.[15] Another effective approach to detect "specificity determining positions" in multiple alignments of subfamily ortholog groups was available in the SDPpred algorithm.[16] The essential results of these analyses are presented in an alignment of pHMM consensus sequences for each of the coronin subfamilies (Fig. 3). Back-shaded residues within the top-line domain sequences denote sites which are conserved but different between subfamily groups, most evident in the multiple aa replacements between coronins 1-4 versus 5-6. Among members of the latter subfamilies, conserved Cys have been replaced by Thr-78 and Gly-152 in coronin 3 and Val-345 in coronin 1. The greatest divergence is seen between the two component halves of coronin 7 sequences, in agreement with the phylogenetic tree (Fig. 1B) and apparent binding and functional differences.[17] Conserved characteristics within each of the three typical WD40 domains can be seen in the HMM logo of Figure 2 although variations between the individual domains and subfamilies can also be discerned, including the presence of a WD dipeptide in the fourth "pseudo" domain despite extensive loss of other WD40 sequence characteristics. Population allelic polymorphisms (e.g., human nsSNPs in Fig. 3) represent another confirmed source of coronin sequence variation.

Corroboration from Genetic Maps and Structures

Exon splicing patterns incorporated into Figure 3 confirm their conservation in species representatives of the individual subfamilies, but marked differences and similarities between subfamilies testify to their relatedness. Only two DUF1900 splice sites are universally conserved, including the split "KGD" motif, whereas marked differences between the monomeric halves of coronin 7 and their use of rare phase-2 introns (i.e., between codon bases 2 and 3) reflect their remote time of divergence. The (dis)similarity between splice sites of coronins 1-4 versus 5-6 reflects the extent of coevolutionary relatedness, with the exception of a coronin 3 WD40 cassette exon splice site, which instead coincides with coronins 5 and 6. It may be noted that total gene lengths, principally reflecting intron sizes, bear only minor resemblance to the evolutionary relatedness of coronins 1, 4 and 6 (all 5-7 kbp), coronins 2 and 3 (both 84 kbp), coronin 7 (62 kbp) and coronin 5 (149 kbp).

The pattern of coronin subfamily expansion near the dawn of vertebrates (Fig. 1A) suggests that it was a consequence of the whole genome duplications believed to have taken place during the chordate to vertebrate transition.[18] Since coronin genes are generally dispersed in vertebrate genomes (see ref. 2) their genetic loci may coincide with the emerging picture of chromosomal duplications being deduced from ongoing genome assemblies. One of the better documented examples of these events comes from the large human "paralogon" groups located on chromosome 9 near band q22.3 (coronin 5 locus) and chromosome 15 in band q23 (coronin 6). We have observed homologous relationships of these same chromosomal regions and the phylogenetic branching between annexins A1 on human chromosome 9q21 and its direct descendent annexin A2 on 15q22.[19] Partial sequences from lamprey and elephant shark strongly suggest their presence in all vertebrate coronin subfamilies, hence their origin from duplication events in the chordate common ancestor. The precise timing of this putative chromosome duplication event involving pairs of coronins, annexins and many other paralogous gene pairs awaits final genome assembly maps for lamprey, hagfish and their chordate predecessors.

3D Modelling of Evolutionary Information

The evaluation of evolutionarily conserved sites for their functional relevance needs to be considered in a realistic spatial context such as 3-dimensional models to distinguish, for example, whether their importance lies in preserving intramolecular protein structure and conformation or in directing intermolecular interactions via external charged residues or surface contours. CONSURF is one of several webservers that employs protein family alignments together with 3D crystal or NMR structural homolog models deposited in the Protein DataBank (http://www.rcsb.org/pdb/) to calculate and display site-specific information about evolutionary conservation.[20] Figure 4 portrays such a model, rendered by MolMol (http://www.mol.biol.ethz.ch/wuthrich/software/molmol/) as a space-filling model of human coronin 4 limited to the backbone atoms of DUF1899, WD40 and DUF1900 domains. The structure is based on the pdb:2aq5 model of mouse coronin 4 (i.e., CORO1A in ref. 7) and the graded shading indicates the level of amino acid conservation at each site based on the entire protein alignment utilized for phylogenetic analysis (Fig. 3). Analytical tools accompanying protein modelling programs assist in molecular inspection by supplying helpful information about solvent accessibility and bond angles and the 3D view offers rotational movement and enhanced visual perspective. The static 2D image in Fig. 4 does however provide some orientative information by localizing the N-terminal basic cluster in DUF1899 on the top surface, the WD dipeptides in WD40 domains comprising part of the propeller scaffold structure at the bottom-right, the highly conserved "KGD" motif in a central, externally exposed region of DUF1900 and part of the C-terminal coiled coil region hidden at the back of the image.

Conclusion

The phylogenetic analysis of known coronins presents a comprehensive overview of this gene family and lays a foundation to advance studies on their distribution, structure and functional diversity in other species. The knowledge of evolutionary relationships should facilitate comparative genomic studies that will help to elucidate the fundamental cellular roles of coronins and rationalize their apparent absence from plants, which are also distinguished by their exceptionally high ratio of monomeric to filamentous actin. The diversity of coronins in unicellular organisms

Molecular Phylogeny and Evolution of the Coronin Gene Family

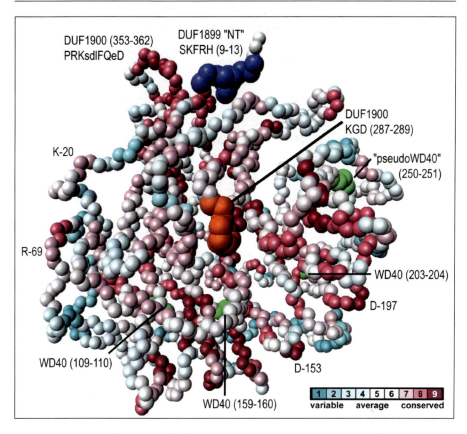

Figure 4. Protein evolution model of human coronin 4 (CRN4, CORO1A). The structure was based on that of the mouse ortholog (pdb:2aq5) and the shading scheme (bottom right) reflects the level of amino acid or property conservation at each site in a space-filling model of atoms comprising only the backbone structure. The grades of evolutionary conservation correspond to a typical coronin (i.e., not solely CRN4) computed from a representative alignment of 80 coronins by Consurf (http://consurf.tau.ac.il/indexnextversion.html) and the final 3D image was rendered by MolMol (http://www.mol.biol.ethz.ch/wuthrich/software/molmol/). Some larger, distinctly shaded motifs are identified by amino acid number and domain location for orientation and to identify significant sites such as the basic-DUF1899 (aa 9-13), KGD-DUF1900 (aa 287-289), Asp-153 and the tryptophan residues of WD40 domains (Trp-109, Trp-159, Trp-203 and Trp-250).

is likely to be much more expansive than is presently known and may help to define basic aspects of their multifunctionality in relation to cellular morphology, vesicular trafficking, locomotion and cytokinesis. Although coronin 7 exhibits the greatest evolutionary success in terms of species distribution, hence functional adaptation, the divergence of the six monomeric subfamilies within vertebrates may be more closely associated with vertebrate-specific functions. The precise timing and mechanisms of the duplicative expansion of these six vertebrate coronin subfamilies will be clarified upon completion of the genome assemblies for early chordates, jawless and cartilaginous fishes. The available data provide perspective and rationale for developing a universal nomenclature for the entire coronin family based on a simple, ordered numbering scheme. Vertebrate coronin subfamilies could be enumerated in reverse evolutionary order of their appearance as coronins 1-7, followed by the incorporation of new coronin 8 and 9 subfamilies descended from their invertebrate common ancestors and terminating with three distant subfamilies based on their species distribution in alveolata (coronin 10), fungi and yeasts (coronin 11) and euglenozoa or amoebae (coronin 12).

The development of pHMM statistical models for each of the individual coronin subfamilies is a powerful tool to classify new homologs and to make pairwise comparisons of molecular profiles with the aim of defining the structural basis of functional specificity for each subfamily. The observation that the domain structures of monomeric coronins are congruent and contain unique, conserved sequence domains (largely of unknown function) will facilitate their structural characterization and comparison with other family members by sequence threading of available 3D structures. These approaches will help to define key functional domains and the basis of sub-family differences. For closely related subfamilies, it is equally important to define the functional determinants of gene and protein regulation, which are also amenable to evolutionary analysis by phylogenetic footprinting.

Computational biology and in silico modelling strategies that utilize evolutionary information from comparative genomic studies can facilitate the prediction, validation and inference of concepts and hypotheses useful in the design and conduct of molecular research. The possibilities go far beyond the present study but they should realistically include molecular docking studies to test the feasibility of putative functional interactions of coronins with, for example, actin and components of known regulatory complexes. Experimental verification of the key functional structures in the unique coronin DUF domains would make a particularly valuable contribution to understanding their subcellular localization, physiological roles and mechanisms. Finally, clinical genetic knowledge about phenotype changes involving coronin single nucleotide polymorphisms (SNPs, see Fig. 3) affecting protein expression, structure and function could be validated by population studies such as HapMap (http://www.hapmap.org/) and combined with molecular modelling studies to help elucidate coronin physiological roles and mechanisms and to identify pathological alleles of medical relevance.

Acknowledgements

This work was supported by research grant BFU2007-67876 from the Ministry of Science and Technology of Spain, research grant IB05-128, personnel support from the "Fundación para el Fomento en Asturias de la Investigación Científica Aplicada y la Tecnología" (FICYT) and the "Programa Ramón y Cajal" jointly funded by the European Union, Spanish Ministry of Education and Science and University of Oviedo.

References

1. Rybakin V, Clemen CS. Coronin proteins as multifunctional regulators of the cytoskeleton and membrane trafficking. Bioessays 2005; 27:625-632.
2. Uetrecht AC, Bear JE. Coronins: the return of the crown. Trends Cell Biol 2006; 16:421-426.
3. de Hostos EL. The coronin family of actin-associated proteins. Trends Cell Biol 1999; 9:345-350.
4. Hussey PJ, Allwood EG, Smertenko AP. Actin-binding proteins in the Arabidopsis genome database: properties of functionally distinct plant actin-depolymerizing factors/cofilins. Phil Trans R Soc Lond B 2002; 357:791-798.
5. Tamura K, Dudley J, Nei M et al. MEGA4: Molecular Evolutionary Genetics Analysis (MEGA) software version 4.0. Mol Biol Evol 2007; 24:1596-1599.
6. Ronquist F, Huelsenbeck JP. MRBAYES 3: Bayesian phylogenetic inference under mixed models. Bioinformatics 2003; 19:1572-1574.
7. Vinh LS, von Haeseler A. IQPNNI: Moving fast through tree space and stopping in time. Mol Biol Evol 2004; 21:1565-1571.
8. Appleton BA, Wu P, Wiesmann C. The crystal structure of murine coronin-1: a regulator of actin cytoskeletal dynamics in lymphocytes. Structure 2006; 14:87-96.
9. Eddy SR. Profile hidden Markov models. Bioinformatics 1998; 14:755-763.
10. Schuster-Bockler B, Schultz J, Rahmann S. HMM logos for visualization of protein families. BMC Bioinformatics 2004; 5(7).
11. Oku T, Itoh S, Okano M et al. Two regions responsible for the actin binding of p57, a mammalian coronin family actin-binding protein. Biol Pharm Bull 2003; 26:409-416.

12. Cai L, Holoweckyj N, Schaller MD et al. Phosphorylation of coronin 1b by protein kinase C regulates interaction with Arp2/3 and cell motility. J Biol Chem 2005; 280:31913-31923.
13. Rosentreter A, Hofmann A, Xavier CP et al. Coronin 3 involvement in F-actin-dependent processes at the cell cortex. Exp Cell Res 2007; 313:878-895.
14. Morgan RO, Martin-Almedina S, Garcia M et al. Deciphering function and mechanism of calcium-binding proteins from their evolutionary imprints. Biochim Biophys Acta—MCR 2006; 1763:1238-1249.
15. Söding J. Protein homology detection by HMM-HMM comparison. Bioinformatics 2005; 21:951-960.
16. Kalinina OV, Mironov AA, Gelfand MS et al. Automated selection of positions determining functional specificity of proteins by comparative analysis of orthologous groups in protein families. Protein Sci 2004; 13:443-456.
17. Rybakin V, Gounko NV, Spate K et al. Crn7 interacts with AP-1 and is required for the maintenance of Golgi morphology and protein export from the Golgi. J Biol Chem 2006; 281:31070-31078.
18. Panopoulou G, Poustka AJ. Timing and mechanism of ancient vertebrate genome duplications—the adventure of a hypothesis. Trends Genetics 2005; 21:559-567.
19. Fernandez MP, Morgan RO. Structure, function and evolution of the annexin gene superfamily, In: Bandorowicz-Pikula J Ed. Annexins: biological importance and annexin-related pathologies, Landes Bioscience/Kluwer Academic/Plenum 2003, pp. 21-37.
20. Glaser F, Pupko T, Paz I et al. ConSurf: identification of functional regions in proteins by surface-mapping of phylogenetic information. Bioinformatics 2003; 19:163-164.

CHAPTER 5

Coronin Structure and Implications

Bernadette McArdle and Andreas Hofmann*

Abstract

Until recently, structural information about coronins was scarce and the earlier identification of five WD40 repeats gave rise to a structural prediction of a five-bladed β propeller for the N-terminal domain of these proteins. More detailed analyses revealed the presence of seven WD40 repeats and the hypothesis of a seven-bladed β propeller structure. This model has recently been validated due to structural information from crystal structures of C-terminally truncated coronin 1 (1A), as well as its C-terminal coiled coil domain. Further structural information is available only indirectly from binding and functional studies.

Phosphorylation at distinct serine and tyrosine residues seems to be a common theme for various coronins. There are indications that this modification regulates the quaternary structure of coronin 3 (1C) and thus has implications for the cellular localisation and the general link between signalling and cytoskeletal remodelling. Similarly, phosphorylation-dependent sorting sequences recently discovered on coronin 7 might prove important for the molecular mechanisms of the longer coronins.

A matter that will require further clarification is the localisation of protein binding sites on coronins. While earlier reports presented a rather diverse map of actin binding sites, more recent studies, including the crystal structure of the coronin 1 N-terminal domain, deliver more detailed information in this respect. Interaction sites for other target proteins, such as Arp2/3, remain to be identified. Also, while membrane binding is a known feature of coronins, further details as to the binding sites and molecular level events remain to be elucidated. The N-terminal WD40 repeat domain seems to be the membrane-interacting domain, but other domains might provide regulatory effects, most likely by posttranslational modification, in a fashion that is specific for each coronin.

In this chapter, we provide a structural overview of coronins 1 (1A), 2 (1B), 3 (1C) and 7 and also present results of our recent efforts to obtain structural models of coronins 3 and 7. Possible implications of these models on the function of these proteins are discussed.

Introduction

Members of the family of coronin proteins are important for the downregulation of the Arp2/3 complex activity that controls F-actin assembly. Functional work so far has concentrated mainly on coronins 1 (1A), 2 (1B) and 3 (1C) and a significant amount of data has been accumulated yielding first insights into localisation and cellular functions of coronins.

While there are two incomplete nomenclatures used in the literature, either differentiating three subclasses of coronins,[1] or a numbering scheme from 1 to 7,[2] we have arbitrarily chosen to use the latter scheme for the purpose of this review. Based on amino acid sequence lengths, coronins can be divided into two classes. Coronins 1-6 are comprised of three domains, whereas mammalian coronin

*Corresponding Author: Andreas Hofmann—Structural Chemistry, Eskitis Institute for Cell and Molecular Therapies, Griffith University, Brisbane Innovation Park, Don Young Road, Brisbane, Qld, 4111, Australia. Email: a.hofmann@griffith.edu.au

The Coronin Family of Proteins, edited by Christoph S. Clemen, Ludwig Eichinger and Vasily Rybakin. ©2008 Landes Bioscience and Springer Science+Business Media.

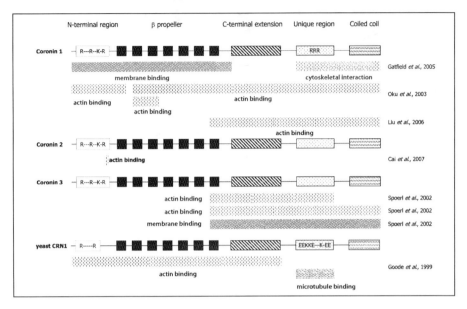

Figure 1. Domain organisation of coronins. Mapped binding sites for yeast coronin (crn1p), as well as mammalian coronins 1 (1A), 2 (1B) and 3 (1C) are indicated.

7 and the POD-1 proteins from *Caenorhabditis elegans* and *Drosophila melanogaster* seem to represent tandem repeats of the short coronin topology.[2] The three-domain topology (see Fig. 1) comprises an N-terminal domain containing WD40 repeats, a linker domain consisting of a C-terminal extension and a unique region, as well as a C-terminal domain that forms a coiled coil structure in some members of the family. Initially, the N-terminal domain was thought to consist of five WD40 repeats.[3] The β subunit of G proteins is the "prototype" WD40 repeat protein and, accordingly, the structure of a five-bladed β propeller has been anticipated for coronins. More recent molecular modelling efforts, however, suggested that seven WD40 repeats might be encoded in the N-terminal domain and the first structure of a coronin N-terminal domain by Appleton and coworkers confirmed this hypothesis.[4] Preceding the WD40 repeat region is a rather short coronin signature motif composed of a dodeca-peptide with conserved basic residues (see Fig. 2, 3).[2] The N-terminal domain is followed by the C-terminal extension and a unique region that differs in length and sequence among different coronins. The C-terminal domain is constituted by a moderately conserved coiled coil, which is of the leucine zipper type in coronin 1 (1A). The coiled coil domain is responsible for homo-oligomerisation observed with several coronin proteins.

This chapter will discuss the structural aspects of coronins and possible implications for its molecular functions. Structural information about coronins is in high demand and the recent crystal structure of a coronin 1 (1A) construct allowed first valuable insights into the building principles and three-dimensional organisation of coronins. However, as with many proteins involved in complex pathways, further structural details are required to dissect and understand the molecular workings and interactions with target proteins. Therefore, this chapter is also a reflection of "work in progress" and some new results from molecular modelling are presented.

WD Repeat

The WD repeat motif has first been identified in the β subunit of the GTP-binding protein transducin and been referred to as transducin repeat, GH-WD repeat, or WD40 repeat.[5-7] A single WD repeat comprises a peptide sequence of 44-60 residues length. The canonical repeat ends with the W-D motif and possesses a G-H sequence about 11-24 residues from its N-terminus.[6] This

```
N-TERMINUS
coronin1   MSRQVVRSSKFRH                                                                    13
coronin3   MRVVVRQSKFRH                                                                     12
pred       CCCCEEEECCCC                    *
coronin7a  MNRFRVSKFRH  TEARPPRRESWISDIRAGTAPSCRNHIKSSC                                      42
pred       CCCCCCCCEEC  CCCEECCCCCCCCCCCCCCEEECCCCCCCC

STRAND     |--A--|              |-B--|          |-C--|       |-D--|
                                                                         *
coronin1                                        VFG          QPAKAD  QCYEDVRVS      31    Blade 7
coronin3                                        VFG          QAVKND  QCYDDIRVS      30
pred                                            CCC          CCCCCC  CCCCCEEE
coronin7b                                                    RDSHIT  NLKGLNLTT      497
pred                                                         CCCCCC  CCCCEEEE

coronin1   QTTWD  SGFCAVN  PK   FMALIC  EASGGG  AFLVLP  LGKTGRVD  KNV   PLVC        78    Blade 1
coronin3   RVTWD  SSFCAVN  PR   FVAIII  EASGGG  AFLVLP  LHKTGRID  KSY   PTVC        77

pred       ECCCC  CEEEEEC  CC   CCCEEE  EECCCC  EEEEEE  CCCCCCCC  CCE   EEEE
coronin7a  KFRHA  QGTVLH        SLIAFN  SDRPG   VLGIVP  LQGQGE D  KRR   VAHL        73
pred       CCCCC  CCEEEE         CEEEEE  CCCCC   EEEEEE  CCCCCC C  CCE   EEEE
coronin7b  PGESD  GFCANK   LR   VAVP    LLSSGG  QVAVLE  LRKPGRLPD TAL   PTLQ        542
pred       CCCCC  CEEEEE   EC   CCCC    EEECCC  CCEEEE  CCCCCCCCC CEE   EEEE

coronin1   GHTAP  VLDIAWC  PHNDN VIASGS  EDC    TVMVWE  IPDGGLVLPL REPV  VTLE       128   Blade 2
coronin3   GHTGP  VLDIDWC  PHNDQ VIASGS  EDC    TVMVWQ  IPENGLTLSL TEPV  VILE       127
pred       ECCCC  EEEEEEC  CCCCC EEEEEC  CCC    EEEEEE  ECCCCCCCCC CCEE  EEEE
coronin7a  GCHSD  LVTDLDF  SPFDDF LLATGS  ADR    TVKLWR  LPGPGQALPS APG   VVL       122
pred       ECCCC  CEEEEEE  CCCCCC EEEEEC  CCC    EEEEEE  ECCCCCCCC  CCE   EEE
coronin7b  NGAA   VTDLAWD  PFDPH  RLAVAG  EDA    RIRLWR  VPAEGLEEVL TTPET VLT       591
pred       CCCC   EEEEEEC  CCCCC  EEEEEC  CCC    EEEEEE  CCCCCCCCCC CCEEE EEE

coronin1   GHTKR  VGIVAWH  PTSQN  VLLSAG  CDN    VILVWD  VGTG      AAV   PTLGPD     173   Blade 3
coronin3   GHSKR  VGIVAWH  PTSRN  VLLSAG  CDN    AIIIWN  VGTG      EAL   INLDD      171
pred       CCCC   EEEEEEC  CCCCC  EEEEE   CCC    EEEEEE  CCCC      CEE   EEEEEC
coronin7a  GPEDL  PVEVLQF  HPTSD  GILVSA  AGT    TVKVWD  AAKQ      QPL   TELA       165
pred       CCCC   EEEEEEE  CCCCC  EEEEE   CCC    EEEEEE  CCCC      CEE   EEEE
coronin7b  GHTEK  ICSLRFH  PLAAN  MLASSS  YDL    TVRIWD  LQAG      ADR   EKLQ       634
pred       CCCC   EEEEEEE  CCCCC  EEEEE   CCC    EEEEEE  CCCC      CEE   EEEE

coronin1   VHPDT  IYSVDKS  RDCA   LICTSC  RDK    RVRVIE  ERKG      TVV   AEKDR      216   Blade 4
coronin3   MHSDM  IYNVSAN  RNGS   LICTAS  KDK    KVRVID  ERKQ      EIV   AEKEK      214
pred       CCCCC  EEEEEEC  CCCC   EEEEEC  CCC    EEEEEE  CCCC      CEE   EEECC
coronin7a  AHGDL  VQSAVKS  RDCA   LVGTA   CKDK   QLRIFD  ERTKP     RAS   QSTQ       208
pred       CCCCC  EEEEEEC  CCCC   EEEE    CCCC   EEEEEE  CCCCC     EEE   EEEE
coronin7b  GHQDQ  IFSLAKS  PDEQ   QLATVC  KDG    RVRVYR  ERSGP     EPL   QEGP       677
pred       CCCCC  EEEEEEC  CCCC   EEEEEC  CCC    EEEEEE  CCCCC     EEE   EEEC

coronin1   PHEGTR PVHAVFV  SEG    KILTTG  FSRMSER QVALWD  TKHLE    EPL   SLQELD     265   Blade 5
coronin3   AHEGAR PMRAIFL  ADG    NVFTTG  FSRMSER QLALWN  PKNMQ    EPI   ALHEMD     263
pred       CCCCCC EEEEEEC  CCC    CEEEEC  CCCCCCC EEEEEE  CCCCC    CEE   EEEECC
coronin7a  AHENSR DSRLAWM  GTWE   HLVSTG  FNQMRER EVKLWD  TRFFSSA  L     ASLTLD     258
pred       CCCCCE EEEEEEC  CCCC   EEEEEE  CCCCCCC EEEEEE  CCCCCCC  E     EEECCC
coronin7b  GPKGGR GARIVWV  CDGR   CLLVSG  FDsqSER QLLLYE  AEALAGG  PL    AVLGLD     728
pred       CCCCCE EEEEEEC  CCCC   EEEEEE  CCCCCCC EEEEEC  CHHCCCC  EE    EEECCC

coronin1   TSSG   VLLPFFD  PDTN   IVYLCG  KGDS   SIRYFE  ITSEAPF   LHYL  SMF        310   Blade 6
coronin3   TSNG   VLLPFYD  PDTS   IIYLCG  KGDS   SIRYFE  ITDESPY   VHYL  NT         307
pred       CCCC   EEEEEEE  CCCC   EEEEEE  CCCC   EEEEEE  CCCCCEE   EEEE  CC
coronin7a  TSLG   CLVPLLD  PDSG   LLVLAG  KGER   QLYCYR  VVPQQPA   LSPVTQCV          304
pred       CCCC   EEEEEEE  CCCC   EEEEEE  CCCC   EEEEEE  CCCCCCE   EEEEEEEE
coronin7b  VAPS   TLLPSYD  PDTG   LVLLTG  KGDT   RVFLYE  LLPESPF   FLECNSFT          774
pred       CCCC   EEEEEEC  CCCC   EEEEEE  CCCC   EEEEEE  ECCCCCE   EEECCCCC

coronin1   SSKES  QRGMGYM  PKRGLEENKCEIA RFYKLH   ER    KCEPIA  MT     QPAKAD QCYEDVRVS  351 Blade 7
coronin3   FSSKEP QRGMGYM  PKRGLDNKCEIA  RFFKLH   ER    KCEPII  MT     QAVKND QCYDDIRVS  349
pred       CCCCCC EEEEEEC  CCCCCEEECCCCC CEEEE    EC    CCCEEE  EE     CCCCCC CCCCCEEE
coronin7a  LESV   LRGAALV  PRQALAMGCE                  VLRVLQ  LSDT   AIVPIGYH         344
pred       CCCC   EEEEEEE  CHHHEEEECCC                 EEEEEE  CCCC   EEEEEEEE
coronin7b  SPDP   HKGLVLL  PKTECDVREVSLM RCLRLR   QSS   LEPVAF  RLP    RDSHIT NLKGLNLTT  816
pred       CCCC   EEEEEEE  CCCCEEEBCCCEE EEEEE    CCC   EEEEEE  BCC    CCCCCC CCCCEEEE

C-TERMINAL EXTENSION / LINKER
coronin1   VPGKEDFTERLKPPTAGPD-PALTAEEALGGRDAGPLLISLKDGYVPPSRELRVNR--GLDS---ARRRATPEPSGTPSSDT-V  430
coronin3   VPSKEDFSDFLAPDTAGPE-AALEAEEAFEGKNADPILISLKHGYIPGKNRDLKVVKNILDSKPTANKKCDLISIPKKTTDTASV   435
pred       BCCCCEEEEEBCCCCCCCC-CCCCHHHHCCCCCEEEEECCCCCCCCCCCCCCCCCEEECCCCCCCCCCCCCCCCCCCCCCC
coronin7a  VPGKAVFHEGLFPDTAGCV-PATDPHGAWAGDNQQVQKVSLNPACRPHPSFTSCLVPPAEPLPDTAQPAVMETPVGDADASEGFSS 430
pred       ECCCCCCCCCCCCCCCCCC-CCCHHHHCCCCCCEEEEECCCCCCCCCCCCCCCCEEECCCCCCCCCCCCCCCCCCCCCCCCCC
coronin7b  RVSK-EFFSDEVFPDTAVIMEVPLSAEAALQGtNGQPWLLSLQPPDMSPVSQAPREAPARRAPSSAQYLEEK              887
pred       CCCC-CCCCCCCCCCCCCCCCCHHHHCCCCCCCCCEEEEECCCCCCCCCCCCCCCCCCCCCCCCCCCC

                                               strand I.1.A ?
                                               -----------
coronin7a  PPSSLTSPSTPSSLGPSLSSTSGIGTSPSLRSLQSLLGPSSKFRHAQGTVLH                                  482
pred       CCEEECCCCCCCCCCCCCCCCCEEECCCCCCCEEECCCCCCCCCEEEE

COILED-COIL
coronin1   SRLEED  VRNLNAI  ------  VQKLQER  LDRLEET  VQAK                                  461
coronin3   QNEAKL  DEILKEI  KSIKDT  ICNQDER  ISKLEQQ  -MAKIAA                                474
pred       CCCHHH  HHHHHHH  HHHHHH  HHHCCHH  HHHHHHH  HHHCCC
coronin7b  SDQQKK  EELLNAM  ------  VAKLGNR  EDPLPQD  -SFEGVDEDEWd                           925
pred       CCCCHH  HHHHHHH  ------  HHHHCCC  CCCCCHH  -HCCCCCCCCCC
```

Figure 2. Legend viewed on next page.

Figure 2, opposite page. Structure-based amino acid alignment of coronins 3 (1C) and 7 with coronin 1 (1A). The line under a specific amino acid sequence indicated as 'pred' shows the predicted secondary structure as obtained by PSIPRED (H – helical, E – extended/β-strand, C – coil).[47] Residues in italics indicate that they provide a structural feature at this location, but appear elsewhere in the amino acid sequence. The residues of the extended coronin signature motif are highlighted by underscore. Arg30, the residue crucial for F-actin bundling in coronin 2 (1B) is marked with *. White on black highlights indicate residues involved in anchoring Trp379 (coronin 1) to the β propeller, white on grey highlights indicate residues involved in the interface around Tyr364 (coronin 1). Conservative mutations in these interfaces are highlighted in grey. The putative phosphorylation site Ser463 (coronin 3) is highlighted by vertical stripes. Shown in bold letters is the acidic motif conserved in all long coronins and similar to those found in Arp2/3-activating proteins of the SCAR/WASP family. The horizontally striped backgrounds indicate the sorting signal recognised by the μ subunit of clathrin assembly protein 1. The very C-terminal region of coronin 7b appears under the 'coiled coil' region simply for purposes of amino acid alignment. Residues 472-482 of coronin 7a might provide strand A of blade 1 of coronin 7a. A color version of this figure is available at www.Eurekah.com.

'structural tetrad' engages in side chain-mediated hydrogen bonding patterns, thereby stabilising the fold. Between the G-H and the W-D motifs, a conserved core sequence has been identified. Hydrophobic residues in this conserved sequence contribute to the stability of the overall fold by van der Waals-interactions between adjacent blades. WD repeat sequences form a secondary structure motif of four consecutive β-strands (D, A, B, C), connected by loops and turns. Crystal structures of the β subunits of G proteins define the prototype WD40 protein structures as β propellers.[8,9] Within the propeller, the blades are arranged in a circular fashion around a central axis. Each blade is made up by four anti-parallel β-strands extending from the centre of propeller to the periphery. Structurally, strand A forms the first and innermost β-strand of a blade. The outermost strand D is provided by the first strand of the next WD repeat.

Earlier Predictions

Earlier structure predictions with coronins resulted in models of five-bladed β propellers, because only five WD repeats were recognised.[3,10] However, many β propeller structures contain WD repeats with little or no obvious sequence homology to the canonical sequence. Additionally, while typical WD repeats possess four to eight copies and up to 16 copies have been reported,[11,12] almost all structures of WD repeat proteins in the PDB contain seven blades per propeller. Keeping this in mind, more detailed analyses of coronins have been carried out and additional WD-like repeats were identified based on secondary structure prediction from amino acid sequences, indicating the presence of seven copies for coronins 1(1A)[13,14] and 3 (1C)[14] and 14 for coronin 7.[14] The fold of a seven-bladed propeller was then confirmed by the crystal structure of a coronin 1 (1A) fragment.[4]

Overall, the WD repeats of coronins show substitutions for the canonical W-D of the structural tetrad, such as Y-E, F-D, L-E, I-E, I-D or W-N. While these substitutions can be considered conservative, others, such as W-R, Y-R or L-R, present a change of electrostatics. Other substitutions such as I-I or I-A seem far off the W-D motif.

Experimental Structures: Coronin 1 N-Terminal and Middle Domain

The first structural information for a coronin construct consisting of the N-terminal domain and the C-terminal extension became available with the crystal structure of coronin 1 (1A) by Appleton and coworkers.[4] Interestingly, despite expressing the full-length murine coronin 1 (1A) in a eukaryotic expression system, these authors found the protein to be proteolytically degraded thus yielding a construct that lacked the C-terminal coiled coil domain. The crystal structure revealed a seven-bladed β-propeller topology for the N-terminal WD repeat domain and a C-terminal domain tightly packed against the bottom side of the propeller. The D strand of blade 7 is provided by the N-terminal residues 17 to 31. Despite the structural tetrad being strictly conserved in blades 2 and

```
N-TERMINUS                                  *
coronin7a  MNRFRVSKFRHTEARPPRRESWISDIRA                                                28
pred       CCCCCCCCEECCCCEECCCCCCCCCCCC
struct     cccceecc eeeeee ccccc
AIP-1      MSEFSQT ALFPSL PRTAR                                                        18
                   |----| -----
                   strand II.7D

STRAND     |--A--|            |-B--|      |-C--|          |-D--|
coronin7a  GTA  PSCRNH IKSSC   SLIAFN SDRPG VLGIVP LQGQGEDKR RVAHL       73  Blade I.1
pred       CCC  EEECCC CCCCC   CEEEEE CCCCC EEEEEE CCCCCCCCC EEEEE
struct     cc   eeeeee ccccc   eeeeee ccc   eeeee  cccccc    eeeee
AIP-1      GT   AVVLGN TPAGD   KIQYCN GTS   VYTVP  VGSLTD    TEIYT      56

coronin7a  GCHSD LVTDLDF SPFDDF LLATGS ADR   TVKLWR LPGPGQALPS APGVVL   122  Blade I.2
pred       ECCCC CEEEEEE CCCCCC EEEEEC CCC   EEEEEE ECCCCCCCCC CCEEEE
struct     ccccc eeeeee  cccc-c eeeeee ccc   ceeeee cccccee    eeeeee
AIP-1      EHSHQ TTVAKT  SPSG-Y YCASGD VHG   NVRIWD TTQTTHI    LKTTIP   100

coronin7a  GPEDL PVEVLQF HPTSD  GILVSA AGT   TVKVWD AAKQQ      PLTELA   165  Blade I.3
pred       CCCCC EEEEEEE CCCCC  EEEEEE CCC   EEEEEE CCCCC      EEEEEE
struct     ccccc eeeeeec cccc   eeeeee ccccc eeeeeecc ccc      eeeeee
AIP-1      VFSGP VKDISWD SESK   RIAAVG EGRER FGHVFLFD TGT      SNGNLT   144

coronin7a  AHGDL VQSAVW SRDGA   LVGTA  CKDK  QLrIFD PRTKP      RASQSTQ  208  Blade I.4
pred       CCCCC EEEEEE CCCCC   EEEEE  CCCC  EEEEEE CCCC       EEEEEEE
struct     ccccc eeeeee ccccc   eeeeee cccc  eeeeee cccc       eeeeee
AIP-1      GQARA MNSVDF KPSRP   FRIISG SDDN  TVAIFE GPPF       KFKSTF   186

coronin7a  AHENS RDSRLAW MGTWE  HLVSTG FNQMRER EVKLWD TRFFSSA  LASLT    256  Blade I.5
pred       CCCCC EEEEEEE CCCCC  EEEEEE CCCCCCC EEEEEE CCCCCCC  EEEEE
struct     cccccc eeeeee ccccc  eeeeee cccc    eeeee  ccccc    eeeeee  ccccccc
AIP-1      GEHTKF VHSVRY NPDGS  LFASTG GDGT    IVLYN  GVDGT    KTGVFE  DDSLKNV  236

coronin7a  LDTSLG CLVPLLD PDSG  LLVLAG KGER  QLYCYE VVPQQP     ALSPVTQCV  304 Blade I.6
pred       CCCCCC EEEEEEE CCCC  EEEEEE CCCC  EEEEEE CCCCCC     EEEEEEEEE
struct     ccccc  eeeeee  cccc  eeeeee ccc   ceeeee ccccc      eeeeee
AIP-1      AHSGS  VFGLTW  SPDGT KIASAS ADK   TIKIWN VATL       KVEKTIP   278

coronin7a  LESV LRGAALV PRQA    LAVM  GCE    VLRVLQ LSDT       AIVPIGYHV 345 Blade I.7
pred       CCCC EEEEEEE CHHH    EEEE  CCC    EEEEEE CCCC       EEEEEEEEE
struct     cccccc eeeeeee cccc  eeeeee ccc   eeeeee ccccc      eeeeee
AIP-1      VGTRIE DQQLGII WTKQ  ALVSIS ANG   FINFVN PELGS      IDQVRY    321

C-TERMINAL EXTENSION
coronin7a  PRKAVEFHEDLFPDTAGCVPATDPHGWWAGDNQQVQKVSLNPACRPHPSFTSCLVPPAEPLPDTAQPAVMETPVGDADASEGFSS  430
pred       CCCCCCCCCCCCCCCCCCCCCCCCHHHHHCCCCCEEEEEECCCCCCCCCCCCCCCCEECCCCCCCCCCCCCCCCCCCCCCC

LINKER
coronin7a  PPSSLTSPSTPSSLGPSLSSTSGIGTSPSLRSLQSLLGPSSKFRHAQGTVLHRDSHITNLKGLNLTTP           498
pred       CCCEECCCCCCCCCCCCCCCCCCEEECCCCCCCEEECCCCCCCCCCCEEEECCCCCCCCCCCEEEEEC

STRAND     |--A--|              |-B--|     |-C--|           |-D--|
coronin7b  GESDQ FCANKL RVAVP    LLS   SGGQV AVLE LRKPGRLPDT ALPTLQ  N      543  Blade II.1
pred       CCCCC EEEEEE CCCCC    EEE   CCCCC EEEE CCCCCCCCCC EEEEEE  C
struct     CCCCC EEEEEE CCCCC    EEEEEE CCCC EEEE CCCCC      EEEEEE  C
AIP-1      GHNKA ITALSS SADGK    TLFSAD AEG  HINSWD ISTGI    SNRVPF  D      364

coronin7b  GAA  VTDLAW DPFDPH    RLAVA  GEDA RIRLWR VPAEGLEEVLTT  PETVLT   591  Blade II.2
pred       CCCC EEEEEE CCCCCC    EEEE   CCCC EEEEEE CCCCCCCCCCCC  EEEEEE
struct     CCCCC EEEEEE CCCCC    EEEE   CCCC EEEEE  CCCCCCCC      EEEEEEE
AIP-1      VHATM ITGIKT TSKGD    LFTVS  WDDH LKVVP  AGGSGVDS      SKAVANKL 410

coronin7b  GHTEK ICSLRW HPLAAN   VLASSS YDL  TVRIWD LQAGA    DRLKLQ          634  Blade II.3
pred       CCCCC EEEEEE CCCCCC   EEEEEE CCC  EEEEEE CCCCC    EEEEE
struct     CCCCC EEEE   CCCCC    EEEEEE CC   EEEEE  CCC      EEEEE
AIP-1      SSQPL GLAV   SAGD     IAVAAC YK   HIAIYS HGK      LTEVP          446

coronin7b  GHQDQ IFSLAW SPDGQ    QLATV  CKDG RVRVYR PRSGP    EPLQEG  P       677  Blade II.4
pred       CCCCC EEEEEE CCCCC    EEEE   CCCC EEEEEE CCCCC    EEEEEE  C
struct     CCCC  EEEEEE CCCCC    EEEEEE CCCC EEEEEE CCCCC    EEEEEEEE CC
AIP-1      ISYN  SSCVAL SNDKQ    FVAVGG QDS  KVHVYK LSGAS    VSEVKTIV HP     491

coronin7b  GPKGG RGARIVW VCDGR   CLLVSG FDsqSER QLLLYE AEALAGG PLAVL        725  Blade II.5
pred       CCCCC EEEEEEE CCCCC   EEEEEE CCCCCCC EEEEEC CHHCCCC EEEE
struct     CC    EEEEEE  CCCCC   EEEEEE CCCC    EEEEE  CCCCC   EEEEEEEEE
AIP-1      AE    ITSVAF  SNNGA   FLVATD QSRK    VIPYS  VANNF   ELAHTNSWT   533

coronin7b  GLDVAPS TLLPSY DPDTG  LVLLTG KGDT RVFLYE LLPESP    FFLE    CNS    772  Blade II.6
pred       CCCCCCC EEEEEE CCCCC  EEEEEE CCCC EEEEEE ECCCCC    EEEE    CCC
struct     CCCCC   EEEEEE CCCCC  EEEEEE CCCC EEEEE  CCCCC    EEEEEEEE
AIP-1      FHTAK   VACVSW SPDNV  RLATGS LDNS VIVWN  MNKPS    DHPIIIKG       577

coronin7b  FTSPDP HKGLVL LPKTE   CDVR   EVE  LMRCLRLR QSS    LEPVAFR  LP    816  Blade II.7
pred       CCCCCC EEEEEE CCCCC   EEEE   CCC  EEEEEEEE CCC    EEEEEEE  CC
struct     CCCCCC EEEEEE CCCCC   EEEEEE CCCC EEEEEE   CCC    eeeeee   ccccc
AIP-1      AHAMS  SVNSVIW LNET   TIVSAG QDSN IKFWN    VPF    ALFPSL   PRTAR 611 (18)

C-TERMINAL EXTENSION
coronin7b  RVRKEFFQDDVFPDTAVWEPVLSAEAWLQGTNGQPWLLSLQPPDMSPVSQAPREAPARRAPSSAQYLEEK         887
pred       CCCCCCCCCCCCCCCCCCCCCCCCHHHHHCCCCCCEEEECCCCCCCCCCCCCCCCCCCCCCC

coronin7b  SDQQKKEELLNAMVAKLGNREDPLPQDSFEGVDEDEWD                                        925
pred       CCCCHHHHHHHHHHHHCCCCCCCHHHCCCCCCCCCC
```

Figure 3. Legend viewed on following page.

Figure 3, opposite page. Structure-based amino acid alignment of coronin 7 with AIP-1, a protein containing two WD domains. Each domain forms a seven-bladed β propeller.[48] The line under a specific amino acid sequence indicated as 'pred' shows the predicted secondary structure as obtained by PSIPRED.[47] The line marked 'struct' shows the secondary structure according to the crystal structure of AIP-1. Abbreviations are the same as in Figure 2. Residues of the coronin signature motif are highlighted by underscore. Arg30, the residue crucial for F-actin bundling in coronin 2 (1B) is marked with *. The horizontally striped highlights indicate the sorting signal recognised by the μ subunit of clathrin assembly protein 1. Shown in grey are residues that have been identified in AIP-1 as crucial for actin disassembly.

3 only, blades 2 to 6 also possess secondary structures that fit the requirements of the β propeller fold. These blades also correspond to the predicted five WD repeats of coronin 1. Blades 1 and 7 are rather atypical in that their W-D motif is substituted by L-P and I-A and their fold shows some divergence from the standard blade. In blade 1, some residues that normally form strand D bulge out and connect to strand C with β-type interactions only at two positions. The D strand of blade 7 consists of two β-strands due to an insertion of six amino acids with a single helical turn in the connecting linker. Some variations in the lengths of strands B and C of blade 7 further add to the structural divergence of this blade from the standard WD40 blade.

It has been known for some time that coronins possess two stretches of conserved amino acid sequence in the C-terminal extension. In the case of coronin 1 (1A), these regions span residues 353-367 and 372-387. The structure by Appleton and coworkers[4] highlighted the distinct roles of the highly conserved residues of Tyr364 and Trp 379. Both residues anchor their side chains into hydrophobic pockets on opposite sides of the bottom surface of the N-terminal β propeller domain, thus stabilising the fold of the C-terminal extension. This domain adopts a rather unstructured conformation and packs against the β propeller due to the high degree of shape complementarity to the N-terminal domain. A network of electrostatic interactions and hydrogen bonds, as well as a hydrophobic interface ensure the strong interactions between both domains.

While there is no structural information on coronin constructs that only contain the N-terminal WD repeat (propeller) domain, severe aggregation has been reported for coronin 1 (1A) truncation mutants lacking the C-terminal extension and the coiled coil domain.[13] The crystal structure of coronin 1 (1A)[4] implies an eminently important role of the C-terminal extension domain for the stability of the protein, especially for the residues directly interacting with the β propeller. Appleton et al.[4] have thus put forward the hypothesis that the region 1-392 of coronin 1 (1A), which comprises the WD repeat domain and the C-terminal extension, represents a folding unit, albeit this awaits experimental validation. Notably, a construct of coronin 3 (1C) extending from the last blade of the β propeller to the coiled coil domain (300-474), possesses secondary structure as predicted and thus appears to be folded.[15] It still remains a matter of speculation, whether blade 7 adopts its native conformation within this construct because strand D is missing.

Experimental Structures: Coiled Coil Peptides

In the context of structural investigation of coiled coil motifs, the group of Steinmetz solved the crystal structure of the mouse coronin 1 (1A) C-terminal coiled coil domain.[16] It is accepted in the field that homo-oligomerisation of coronins is mediated by the C-terminal coiled coil domain. While electron micrographs, as well as analytical ultracentrifugation, showed coronin 1 (1A) homo-trimerisation,[13] prediction programs such as MultiCoil[17] or Scorer[18] suggest two-stranded structures. A study by Oku and coworkers also reported the presence of dimeric coronin 1 (1A) based on gel filtration and sucrose density centrifugation[19] and therefore is at odds with the generally accepted view. It has been suggested that their results might have been biased due to shape-dependency of the methods used.

Coiled coil motifs usually show a characteristic repeat pattern of hydrophobic amino acids spaced four and then three residues apart. This results in a hepta-peptide repeat $(abcdefg)_n$, where positions a and d are predominantly hydrophobic residues and positions e and g are charged residues. Coronin 1 (1A) possesses a threefold repeat of such a characteristic hepta-peptide sequence and the motif R-L/I/V-X-X-L/V-E (450-455 in coronin 1) has been identified as a mediator of trimerisation in coiled coils.[16] The arginine residue (position 1) of one monomer engages in interactions with the glutamate residue (position 6) from a second monomer. The interaction is stabilised by further contacts of this arginine residue (position 1) with an aspartate residue of the second monomer at position 3. Overall, this network of interactions maintains a contact interface of three monomers.

Coronin 3 N-Terminal Domain

Coronin 3 (1C) belongs to the subfamily of the short coronins with a length of 474 amino acids. It is expressed in all tissues and performs roles in wound healing, protrusion formation including lamellipodia, filopodia and axonal growth, migration, invasion, cell proliferation, cytokinesis, endocytosis, secretion of norepinephrine and matrix metalloproteinases.[15,20] Localised to the leading edges of a cell and the sub-membranous cytoskeleton, it acts by bundling F-actin and crosslinking the Arp2/3 complex and cofilin.[15,21,22] Based on the crystal structures of coronin 1 (1A) (8-402)[4] and the three-stranded coiled coil domain (430-461),[16] homology models for these domains in coronin 3 (1C) have been generated.[15,23]

Most likely, coronin 3 (1C) seems to exhibit the same feature as coronin 1 (1A) with the first N-terminal β-strand completing the last propeller blade of the WD40 repeat domain.[15] Intra-molecular interactions might stabilise the C-terminal extension by anchoring it to the WD40 β-propeller. The main contributors to these interactions are hydrogen bonds of Tyr362 to the backbone carbonyl groups of Val327 and Glu331 and the side chain interactions of the N-terminal Lys9 with Arg352 and Asp360. Between the WD40 repeat domain and the C-terminal extension, there is also a hydrophobic interface comprising residues His139, Ile157, Trp182, Ile189 and Trp377 and Phe378. The high degree of conservation between both coronins in these regions underpins the potential significance of these interactions. The potential F-actin binding sites identified in coronin 1 (1A)[4] seem highly probable in coronin 3 (1C), including a region on the top of blades 1, 6, 7 and a second region on the bottom side of blades 6 and 7. A stretch of positively charged amino acids is also present in the C-terminal extension (398-419).[15]

An amino acid alignment of coronin 3 (1C) and coronin 1 (1A) generated before these models have been available, identified the peptide of 308-349 as seventh WD40 repeat[14] and gave rise to two truncation mutants comprising peptides spanning (i) the last WD40 repeat and the entire C-terminal part of coronin 3 (300-474) and (ii) the last WD40 repeat and the C-terminal extension domain (315-444). CD spectra for both constructs show the of secondary structure as expected from structure prediction.[15]

An interesting observation in this context is the fact that these truncation mutants of coronin 3 seem to adopt functional structures. Both constructs have been shown to bind, bundle and crosslink F-actin in in vitro studies. The same activity has been found with coronin 3 (300-474), the construct described above.[21,22]

Coronin 3 Coiled Coil Domain: Effects of Phosphorylation

The extreme C-terminal region of coronin 3 (1C) is eight residues longer than that of coronin 1 (1A) and secondary structure prediction indicates a long helical segment (see Fig. 2). Furthermore, coronin 3 (1C) possesses a fourfold repeat of the characteristic coiled coil hepta-peptide sequence. Using the programme MultiCoil,[17] the C-terminal domain of coronin 3 (1C) is predicted to form mainly homo-trimers (60% probability), but also homo-dimers (18% probability). Homo-trimers have also been observed in vitro.[21]

Using the crystal structure of the coronin 1 (1A) coiled coil trimer (PDB entry 2akf)[16] and molecular graphics, a model of the three-stranded coronin 3 (1C) coiled coil has been generated.[23] Like coronin 1 (1A), coronin 3 (1C) possesses the characteristic hexa-peptide motif R-L/I/V-X-X-L/V-E (461-466) proposed to be regulating trimerisation of coiled coil strands. Notably, while coronin 1 has Asp452 in position 3 of this motif, coronin 3 (1C) possesses Ser463 instead. Ser463 is a predicted phosphorylation site and the addition of a phosphate group to this residue will lead to disruption of the Arg461'-Glu466 interaction. Phosphorylation will require displacement of the Arg461' side chain and thus lead to the loss of the one of the coils. The remaining two-stranded coiled coil is probably stabilised by interactions arising from the reoriented Arg461' side chain and possibly bridging effects from the posttranslational modification. Ser450 is part of a hexa-peptide insertion in coronin 3 (1C) that is not present in the coronin 1 (1A) coiled coil and can potentially be phosphorylated as well. While a role of (phosphorylated) Ser450 for di-/trimerisation cannot be excluded, it seems unlikely as judged by the current homology model. Ser450 is purely surface-exposed and does not seem to be involved in strategic interactions.

This mechanism is supported by results from gel filtration experiments with the phosphomimetic mutant Ser463Asp of a coronin 3 (1C) C-terminal peptide, as well as the full-length protein, which elute as a dimeric species. The wild type peptide and protein, in contrast, elute as a trimer in the size exclusion experiments.[23] Also, phosphorylation at Ser463 regulates the oligomerisation state of coronin 3 (1C) and subsequently alters its cellular activity.

While phosphorylation of coronin 3 (1C) has been found to be correlated with its cytosolic location,[21] cytosolic coronin 7 is not phosphorylated; the membrane-associated pool of coronin 7, however, is phosphorylated at tyrosine residues.[24] A similar situation is found with coronin 1, where dissociation from phagocytotic vacuoles is dependent on the protein being phosphorylated.[25] For coronin 2 (1B), a partial redistribution from vesicular structures to the leading edge of actin-rich filopodia has been reported upon phosphorylation by PKC on Ser2, a residue present in coronin 1 (1A), but not coronins 3 (1C) and 7.[26,27] The modification also disrupts the interaction of the protein with the Arp2/3 complex.

Actin Binding Site

Actin binding can be considered the landmark features of coronins as they are collectively defined as F-actin-associated proteins.[3] The common theme appears to be that coronins possess an actin binding site in the C-terminal domain, although further details remain to be clarified (see Fig. 1). For coronin 3 (1C), constructs comprising the last WD40 repeat and the entire C-terminal part, with (315-474) or without (315-444) the coiled coil domain, have been shown to bind and crosslink F-actin.[21] Different studies for mammalian coronin 1 (1A) agree on the finding that the C-terminal part possesses a binding site for actin.[13,28,29] The smallest common region in this context has been described by Gatfield and coworkers to be the region from 400 to 416 which is in the unique part of the C-terminal domain of coronin 1 (1A) and contains a patch of basic amino acids.[13] Many actin binding proteins use such a feature to form favourable electrostatic interactions with acidic regions on F-actin.[30,31] Oku and coworkers have also described actin-binding properties of peptides in the N-terminal domain of mammalian coronin 1 (1A), namely the very N-terminal region (signature motif) and a region spanning propeller blades 2 and 3.[29] One study concerned with yeast coronin (crn1p) mapped the actin binding property to the N-terminal domain with a peptide spanning the residues 1-400. At the same time, C-terminal constructs of yeast coronin did not show any actin binding behaviour.[32]

The crystal structure of the coronin 1 (1A) N-terminal and C-terminal extension domains provides some insights into the apparent confusion. Appleton and coworkers[4] identified two patches conserved among the short coronins that might be involved in actin binding. One patch is formed by residues from propeller blades 1, 6 and 7 on the top face of the WD40 repeat domain. The other patch is located on the bottom face and is made up by residues from blades 6 and 7, as well as from the C-terminal extension domain.[4]

Very recently, a study concerned with coronin 2 (1B) revealed a crucial role of Arg30 in F-actin binding.[33] Consistent with an important role for interactions between coronin 2 (1B) and F-actin in vivo, an Arg30Asp mutant does not bind F-actin and localises to the leading edge only inefficiently. The authors show that this residue selectively impairs the actin binding step, since interactions with Arp2/3 and others are identical to the wild type protein. An exciting result from co-immunoprecipitation using the Arg30Asp mutant as a tool suggests that it is the actin binding that increases the affinity of coronin 2 (1B) for Arp2/3.[33] Interestingly, Arg30 is part of the coronin signature motif[2] and, accordingly, a homology model of coronin 2 (1B) showing this residue surface-exposed and not involved in any other interactions is presented.[33] The residue is in vicinity of Lys73 and both residues have been shown to impair F-actin bundling. The basic patch on the surface of coronin 2 (1B) can putatively act as actin binding site and the conservation of these residues in coronins 1(1A) and 3 (1C) imply that the other short coronins also possess the same mechanism.

While any detailed model awaits experimental evidence, it is tempting to speculate that two separate actin binding sites could fulfill a role of coronins in F-actin crosslinking. On the other hand, it is still not undoubtedly clear whether the N- and C-terminal domains each harbour an actin binding site or whether one of them (most likely the one on the C-terminal side) acts as a regulatory element. Furthermore, it is not yet proven whether Arg30 in coronin 2 (1B) binds actin directly or actually interacts with the nucleotide.

For coronin 7, actin binding has not been observed to date.[24] While it is difficult to explain this absence on the basis of the available structural models, it seems possible that the two anticipated actin-binding patches identified in the crystal structure of coronin 1(1A) are not accessible in the same way in coronin 7 due to inter-domain contacts between coronin 7a and 7b. Arg30, the residue critical for actin binding in coronin 2 (1B), is conserved in coronin 7a, but not 7b, albeit we hypothesise it to be located in a different structural element (see Figs. 2 and 3). Lys67 in coronin 7a is a conserved lysine residue in coronins 1(1A) and 3 (1C), but not coronin 7b (Thr536) and has also been reported to be involved in actin binding of coronin 2 (1B).[33] The structural localisation of this lysine residue in coronin 7a might be conserved according to available models (Figs. 2 and 3), but this residue might only be functional in actin binding when in close vicinity to Arg30.

Association with Plasma Membrane

To date, no binding partners of coronins at the plasma membrane have been identified. The common function of the β propeller fold of WD repeat proteins is that of a binding platform yielding complexes by coordinating sequential or simultaneous interactions with binding proteins.[6] Because the coiled coil domain is involved in homo-oligomerisation and possibly binding to the Arp2/3 complex (see below) and the C-terminal extension domain might bind F-actin, one could assume that the membrane-associated functions reside on the β propeller domains of coronins. Notably, this might have implications on the N-terminal actin binding site, if the sites of interaction with the membrane are identical or in close vicinity to the actin-binding patch. However, the scenario is supported by the observation that an N-terminal domain construct of coronin 1 (1A) shows plasma membrane binding in the absence of the unique C-terminal and the coiled coil domains (see Fig. 1).[13] One would thus assume that plasma membrane association of coronin 1 does not require a trimeric species, but this remains to be proven by further experimental data. In an earlier study, these authors have suggested that binding partners can include integral and peripheral membrane proteins, as well as phospholipid moieties themselves.[34]

A different situation has been found with coronin 3 (1C), where the deletion of the coiled coil domain abolishes plasma membrane binding.[22] Taking into account the role of the coiled coil domain for homo-oligomerisation and the fact that phosphorylation in this domain can alter the oligomerisation state, a further twist becomes apparent. Phosphorylation of coronin 3 (1C) leads to a cytosolic relocation of coronin 3 (1C), i.e., loss of association with the plasma membrane.[21] One could conclude that the membrane association of coronin 3 (1C) is also mediated by the β propeller domain, but that this only occurs with the trimeric species. In the absence of experimental data, other binding sites in the C-terminal domain of coronin 3 (1C) cannot be excluded, though.

Intra- Versus Inter-Molecular Coronin Interactions

In vivo and in vitro co-immunoprecipitation studies with several coronin 3 (1C) constructs lead to the observation that the N-terminal peptide 1-71 binds to a region in the C-terminal domain (315-444).[21] The site at the C-terminal domain is close to or overlaps with the actin binding site, since markedly reduced F-actin cosedimentation was also observed for certain combinations of coronin 3 (1C) truncation constructs. While the binding was observed as an inter-molecular interaction, it is in principle possible that, physiologically, this is in fact an intra-molecular interaction. In light of the crystal structure of coronin 1 (1A) and the derived models for coronin 3 (1C), there is further weight to the notion that these interactions came about as artefacts from the topology of the different constructs. Because all truncation constructs in that study, as well as in most other coronin studies to date, are sequential, but the β propeller topology is not, it might prove difficult to obtain 'physiological' results with correctly folded peptides. For example, a plausible scenario for an interaction study of coronin 3 (1-72) with coronin 3 (315-444) might be that the N-terminal domain peptide provides a β-strand for completion of the last propeller blade in the C-terminal construct. Obviously, like many other aspects of coronin structure and function, the question of possible coronin interactions other than the coiled coil oligomerisation would benefit from further structural data.

Coronin Protein-Protein Interactions

Apart from F-actin, the Arp2/3 complex has been identified as a binding partner for coronins[35] and the binding site has been mapped to the coiled coil region in yeast coronin (crn1p).[36] Coronin constructs missing the coiled coil domain do not bind to the Arp2/3 complex.[4] Recently, the structure of the yeast Arp2/3 complex has been investigated by electron microscopy and density in a distance of about 20 Å from the core complex has been assigned to the β propeller of coronin.[37] The distance has been explained by the long C-terminal extension domain and unique region of yeast coronin and the arrangement thus fits the model of the coiled coil domain interacting with the complex. The structure also shows that coronin stabilises an inactive conformation of the Arp2/3 complex which agrees with functional data from polymerisation assays, where the protein inhibits the Arp2/3-mediated F-actin nucleation.[37]

Coronin 2 (1B) has also been found to be colocalised with the Arp2/3 complex in a variety of cells.[26] The interaction of coronin 2 with Arp2/3 is phosphorylation-dependent and Ser2, located in the very N-terminal region has been identified as the crucial site of regulation by PKC in this context. Consistent with the functional data from coronin 1 (1A), a nonphosphorylatable mutant of coronin 2 (1B), Ser2Ala, shows enhanced interactions with the Arp2/3 complex and promotes hypermotility in cellular assays to a greater extent than the wild type protein.[26] In line with these findings, the phospho-mimetic Ser2Asp mutant of coronin 2 (1B) displayed weaker interactions with Arp2/3 and suppressed cell speed relative to the wild type.[26] The same findings were obtained with the Ser2Asp mutant of coronin 1 (1A) investigated in a coronin 1 (1A) knock out mouse.[38] The functional paradox of these findings is striking: Coronin acts as a molecular inhibitor of Arp2/3 by stabilising an inactive form of the complex. At the cellular level, however, this turns out to be an activating process for Arp2/3-dependent processes such as cellular motility. Further studies will be required to shine light on these complex interconnections.

Since the Arp2/3 binding site on coronin 2 (1B) is presumably located in the C-terminal region of the protein just like in other coronins, it remains to be clarified which molecular mechanisms are responsible for coupling the modification of Ser2 in the N-terminal region to the Arp2/3 binding site in the C-terminal domain.

Very recently, slingshot phosphatase (SSH1L), a regulator of actin filament formation that acts on ADF/cofilin, has been shown to bind to coronin 2 (1B) simultaneously with the Arp2/3 complex. In a tandem co-immunoprecipitation experiment, Cai and coworkers could demonstrate that all three components are present in one complex and coronin 2 (1B) bridges SSH1L to the Arp2/3 complex.[39] Furthermore, the study shows that coronin 2 (1B) is also a substrate of slingshot phosphatase and the phosphatase seems to be specific for coronin and cofilin in vivo, as no dephosphorylation of other focal adhesion-associated proteins (Erk1/2, paxillin) has been observed. While dephosphorylation and complex formation provide mechanistic details about the inhibitory effect of coronin 2 (1B) on Arp2/3-mediated actin nucleation, another important aspect became apparent in that study. Coronin 2 (1B) seems to target SSH1L to the leading edge of lamellipodia, as well as mediate cofilin activity via dephosphorylation by SSH1L.

Homology Models of Coronin 7

The subfamily of long coronins is constituted by four proteins: POD-1 from *Caenorhabditis elegans*,[40] Dpod-1 from *Drosophila melanogaster*,[41] the mammalian coronin 7,[24] as well as villidin, a long chimeric coronin-like protein.[42] These proteins are about twice as long as their shorter relatives and it is assumed that the corresponding genes arose due to gene duplication. The long coronins contain two copies of the basic coronin domain structure, i.e., two WD repeat domains, two C-terminal extension domains, but both copies lack the coiled coil segments. It is assumed that the dimer character of the long coronins renders further oligomerisation of these proteins unnecessary.[1] The structural and functional significance of the domain organisation in the long coronins remains unknown. For Dpod-1, a microtubule-binding domain has been predicted similar to that of the microtubule-binding protein MAP1B.

Mammalian coronin 7 is the first member of this family that has been localised to the Golgi and is believed to execute membrane trafficking-related functions; however, there is no indication for a Golgi localisation of the worm and fly PODs.[24] In contrast to cytosolic coronin 3 (1C), cytosolic coronin 7 is not phosphorylated. However, the fact that membrane-associated coronin 7 is phosphorylated at tyrosine residues makes it a plausible assumption that the protein relocates from the cytosol to the membrane upon phosphorylation.[24] Two tyrosine-based sorting signals recognised by the μ subunits of clathrin assembly protein 1 (AP-1) have been identified in coronin 7. Peptides containing the Y-X-X-Φ motifs at Tyr288 and Tyr758, respectively, have been found to bind to AP-1 and coronin 7 has been shown to coprecipitate with AP-1.[43] Kinase src binds to coronin 7 and both tyrosines 288 and 758 are specifically phosphorylated by src. Tyrosine 758 however appears as the major phosphorylation site of src, which thus may be a key regulator of coronin 7.[44]

Two different models of coronin 7 structural organisation can be envisioned: One model is based on alignment with coronins 1 (1A) and 3 (1C) (see Fig. 2), the other is based on an alignment with actin-interacting protein 1 (AIP-1; see Fig. 3). AIP-1 is a WD repeat protein that enhances actin filament disassembly in the presence of actin-depolymerising factor/cofilin. The sequence similarities of the two WD40 domains of human AIP-1 with the ones of coronin 7 are about 20%; the sequence similarities with *C. elegans* AIP-1 are 23% and 26%, respectively. We have chosen AIP-1 as a template for modelling coronin 7 structural organisation due to its structure having two β propeller domains in tandem.[45]

Based on the structures of coronin 1 (1A) and AIP-1, the main difference in topologies between the two derived coronin 7 models (see Fig. 4) is the involvement of the most N-terminal β-strand and, subsequently, the first β-strand after the C-terminal extension domain of coronin 7a in the formation of the β propeller structure. When analysing the secondary structure prediction of coronin 7a, β-strand topology is predicted for residues 32-34. One can adopt the view that this is not significant enough to make the first β-strand of blade 1, because all other coronins have a well conserved secondary structure element in this position with a length of four to six residues. A suggestion to reconcile could involve the first β-strand after the C-terminal extension of coronin 7a. The model based on AIP-1, however, makes use of the very N-terminal β-strand, thus not assigning a canonical β propeller function for the β-strand in the linker region between coronin 7a and 7b.

The second ambiguity in predicting a model of the tandem WD40 domains of coronin 7 is the role of the short β-strand in blade 7 of coronin 7b. In homology to coronin 1 (1A), this element would not participate in the canonical blade formation. The model based on AIP-1, on the other hand, makes use of that element which provides strand II.7B (see Fig. 3). Obviously, other combinations can be envisioned. Three secondary structure elements, the most N-terminal β-strand, as well as two β-strands in the linker region, can potentially participate in any of the 14 blades as strand A or D.

In an attempt to learn about the putative conformation of the two β propellers of coronin 7, we compared the fold of AIP-1 (PDB entry 1nr0)[45] with that of another tandem β propeller protein with known three-dimensional structure, namely Sro7 (PDB entry 2oaj).[46] Sro7 is a regulator of

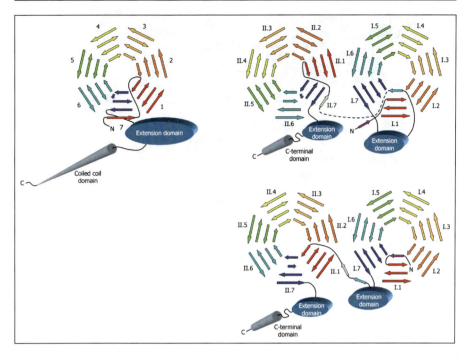

Figure 4. Putative topology of coronins 3 (1C) and 7. Left panel: Based on the structural information for coronin 1 (coronin 1A) and amino acid sequence alignments, a topology for coronin 3 can be proposed that is highly similar to coronin 1. Right panel: Possible topologies for coronin 7 based on a structure-based sequence alignment with coronins 1 and 3 (upper right panel) and with AIP-1 (lower right panel).

polarised exocytosis and interacts with Q-SNARE proteins, thereby coordinating the actin cytoskeleton and the exocytic machinery responsible for fusion of secretory vesicles. The comparison indicates that there is considerable variability in the orientation of the two β propellers in tandem WD40 repeat domain structures (see Fig. 5). In both proteins, blades 7 and 1 of the first propeller are in close proximity to blades 1 and 7 of the second propeller. However, the elevations between the two propeller axes are about 45° for Sro7 and 60° for AIP-1. The azimuth between the two propeller axes is about 15° for Sro7 and –30° for AIP-1. While the two β propellers of the latter protein have several contacts between blades 1 and 7 of both propellers, the smaller elevation angle in Sro7 results in only blade 1 of the first propeller and blade 7 of the second propeller being in close proximity. In both proteins, it is the loop area between strands C and D of blade 1 of the first propeller that interacts with blade 7 of the second propeller. The evident variability of the orientation of propellers in tandem WD40 repeat domain structures adds to the complexity of any modelling endeavours for coronin 7 and calls upon experimental structures for clarification of structural details.

The N-terminal coronin signature motif R-X-X-K-X-R is present in coronin 7a only. The extended signature motif in coronins 1 and 3 of R-X-X-K-X-R-X_7-K-X_8-R finds a pendant in the sequence R-X-X-K-X-R-X_7-R-X_8-R in coronin 7a. While in coronin 1 (1A) this extension is located in strand D of blade 7 and Lys20/Arg29 are accessible on the surface of the propeller, a definite answer as to the location of this motif in coronin 7a cannot be given based on the current models (see Fig. 4). A model where this motif is not surface-accessible in coronin 7a would explain the observation that coronin 7 is not colocalising with actin. While coronin 7a shows a conservation of Arg27 and Lys67 that have been proven crucial for F-actin cable formation in coronin 2 (1B),

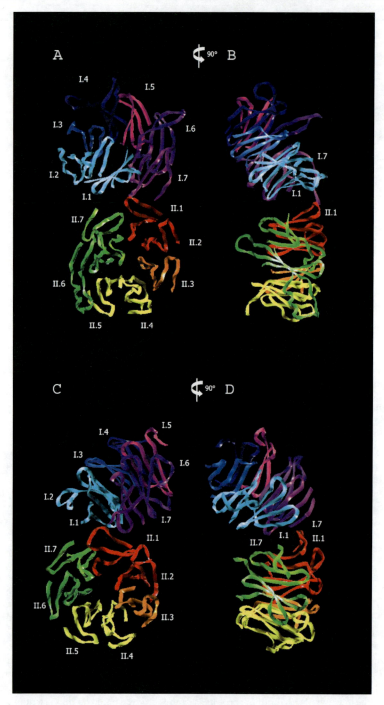

Figure 5. Conformational variation of tandem β propeller structures. Front and side views of the two tandem β propeller structures: Sro7 (PDB entry 2oaj; *A, B*)[46] and AIP (PDB entry 1nr0; *C, D*)[45]. Propeller blades are numbered. Figure prepared with SYBYL (Tripos).

the location of Arg27 is not the same as in coronin 1 (1A), since the N-terminal β-strand is not forming the strand D of the last propeller blade in neither of our two coronin 7 models (see Figs. 2, 3). Lys67, however, might be in the same location but seems to play a less important role in F-actin regulation.[33] Coronin 7b has neither of the two basic residues conserved and is thus unlikely to possess this molecular mechanism.

The alignment of coronin 7 with coronins 1 (1A) and 3 (1C) allows some other interesting observations (see Fig. 2). While coronin 7 is not predicted to form any coiled coil structure, coronin 7b does seem to posses a C-terminal extension domain, albeit smaller than in other coronins. This assumption is based on the conserved helical segment in the linker region following the last propeller blade. Furthermore, the two aromatic residues involved in anchoring the C-terminal extension to the β propeller are conserved in both coronin 7 parts (Phe357, Trp372, Phe828, Trp844). Phe357 and Phe828 would be expected to engage in contacts with a V-X-X-X-E motif in the seventh propeller blade which is also conserved in coronin 7a and 7b, although the mechanism observed in coronin 1 (1A) involves hydrogen bonding from Tyr364 to the backbone carbonyls of Val327 and Glu331. The exchange of the tyrosine residue against a phenylalanine renders this type of interaction obsolete. Other residues involved in formation of this interaction interface are conserved to varying extents in coronin 7a and 7b (white on gray highlighted residues in Fig. 2). Trp379, the second anchor in the linker domain, is actually part of a W-Φ motif also conserved in all coronins 1, 3, 7a and 7b. This residue forms a hydrophobic interaction interface with various residues in blades 3 and 4 of the β propeller. While coronin 7a has several, but not all of these interface residues conserved, coronin 7b shows full conservation (white on black highlighted residues in Fig. 2). Taken together, this would allow the conclusion that an interface similar to that observed in coronin 1 (1A) can be expected for both coronin 7 propellers at the bottom faces.

Conclusion

Based on cell biological studies, as well as the first crystal structure of a coronin 1 (1A) fragment, first insights into structure and mechanisms of coronins have been obtained, mainly pointing out the features of the WD40 repeat domain and the importance of the C-terminal extension for the stability of the former. From a mechanistic point of view, the upcoming main questions are those of oligomerisation, actin binding and the features of coronin 7 which represents a tandem coronin monomer. With the recent identification of Arg30 on coronin 2 (1B) as an important regulator for F-actin bundling, a new tool for further investigation of the actin binding mechanisms of coronins has become available. At the molecular level, the events and localisations in this context remain to be identified. A model for the oligomerisation mechanism of coronin 3 (1C) has been put forward and is currently being validated by cell biological experiments. The area with the highest level of speculation is that of structure-function relationships of the long coronins, such as coronin 7. In this chapter, we have presented two possible models outlining structural parameters of these tandem WD40 repeat domain proteins. Aiding the further proceeding of this field, structural biology will be able to provide insights into the molecular functions of coronins and help define their roles in cell development.

Acknowledgements

AH gratefully acknowledges funding by Griffith University Research Grant, and an award from the European League Against Rheumatism (EULAR).

References

1. Uetrecht AC, Bear JE. Coronins: the return of the crown. Trends Cell Biol 2006; 16:421-426.
2. Rybakin V, Clemen CS. Coronin proteins as multifunctional regulators of the cytoskeleton and membrane trafficking. BioEssays 2005; 27:625-632.
3. de Hostos EL. The coronin family of actin-associated proteins. Trends Cell Biol 1999; 9:345-350.
4. Appleton BA, Wu P, Wiesmann C. The crystal structure of murine coronin-1: a regulator of actin cytoskeletal dynamics in lymphocytes. Structure 2006; 14:87-96.
5. Vander V, Ploegh HL. The WD-40 repeat. FEBS Lett 1992; 307:131-134.

6. Smith TF, Gaitatzes C, Saxena K et al. The WD repeat: a common architecture for diverse functions. Trends Biochem Sci 1999; 24:181-185.
7. Neer EJ, Schmidt CJ, Nambudripad R et al. The ancient regulatory-protein family of WD-repeat proteins. Nature 1994; 371.
8. Wall MA, Coleman DE, Lee E et al. The structure of the G protein heterotrimer $G_{i\alpha 1}\beta_1\gamma_2$. Cell 1995; 83:1047-1058.
9. Lambright DG, Sondek J, Bohm A et al. The 2.0 Angstrom crystal structure of a heterotrimeric G protein. Nature 1996; 379.
10. Suzuki K, Nishihata J, Arai Y et al. Molecular cloning of a novel actin-binding protein, p57, with a WD repeat and a leucine zipper motif. FEBS Lett 1995; 364.
11. Li D, Roberts R. WD-repeat proteins: structure characteristics, biological function and their involvement in human diseases. Cell Mol Life Sci 2001; 58:2085-2097.
12. Yu L, Gaitatzes C, Neer EJ et al. Thirty-plus functional families from a single motif. Protein Sci 2000; 9:2470-2476.
13. Gatfield J, Albrecht I, Zanolari B et al. Association of the leukocyte plasma membrane with the actin cytoskeleton through coiled coil-mediated trimeric coronin 1 molecules. Mol Biol Cell 2005; 16:2786-2798.
14. Clemen CS, Hofmann A. Unpublished.
15. Rosentreter A, Hofmann A, Xavier CP et al. Coronin 3 involvement in F-actin-dependent processes at the cell cortex. Exp Cell Res 2007; 313:878-895.
16. Kammerer RA, Kostrewa D, Progias P et al. A conserved trimerization motif controls the topology of short coiled coils. Proc Natl Acad Sci 2005; 102:13891-13896.
17. Wolf E, Kim PS, Berger B. MultiCoil: a program for predicting two- and three-stranded coiled coils. Prot Sci 1997; 6:1179-1189.
18. Woolfson DN, Alber T. Predicting oligomerization states of coiled coils. Prot Sci 1995; 4:1596-1607.
19. Oku T, Itoh S, Ishii R et al. Homotypic dimerisation of the actin-binding protein p57/coronin-1 mediated by a leucine zipper motif in the C-terminal region. Biochem J 2005; 387:325-331.
20. Thal DR, Xavier C-P, Rosentreter A et al. Expression of coronin 3 in diffuse gliomas is related to malignancy. 2007; submitted.
21. Spoerl Z, Stumpf M, Noegel AA et al. Oligomerization, F-actin interaction and membrane association of the ubiquitous mammalian coronin 3 are mediated by its carboxyl terminus. J Biol Chem 2002; 277:48858-48867.
22. Hasse A, Rosentreter A, Spoerl Z et al. Coronin 3 and its role in murine brain morphogenesis. Eur J Neurosci 2005; 21:1155-1168.
23. Xavier C-P, Rosentreter A, Hofmann A et al. Phosphorylation regulates the quaternary structure and activity of coronin 3. Manuscript in preparation 2007.
24. Rybakin V, Stumpf M, Schulze A et al. Coronin 7, the mammalian POD-1 homologue, localizes to the Golgi apparatus. FEBS Lett 2004; 573:161-167.
25. Itoh S, Suzuki K, Nishihata J et al. The role of protein kinase C in the transient association of p57, a coronin family actin-binding protein, with phagosomes. Biol Pharm Bull 2002; 25:837-844.
26. Cai L, Holoweckyj N, Schaller MD et al. Phosphorylation of coronin 1B by protein kinase C regulates interaction with Arp2/3 and cell motility. J Biol Chem 2005; 280:31913-31923.
27. Parente JA, Chen X, Zhou C et al. Isolation, cloning and characterization of a new mammalian coronin family member, coroninse, which is regulated within the protein kinase C signaling pathway. J Biol Chem 1999; 274:3017-3025.
28. Liu CZ, Chen Y, Sui SF. The identification of a new actin-binding region in p57. Cell Res 2006; 16:106-112.
29. Oku T, Itoh S, Okano M et al. Two regions responsible for the actin binding of p57, a mammalian coronin familz actin-binding protein. Biol Pharm Bull 2003; 26:409-416.
30. Tang JX, Janmey PA. The polyelectrolyte nature of F-actin and the mechanism of actin bundle formation. J Biol Chem 1996; 271:8556-8563.
31. Amann KJ, Renley BA, Ervasti JM. A cluster of basic repeats in the dystrophin rod domain binds F-actin through an electrostatic interaction. J Biol Chem 1998; 273:28419-28423.
32. Goode BL, Wong JJ, Butty AC et al. Coronin promotes the rapid assembly and cross-linking of actin filaments and may link the actin and microtubule cytoskeletons in yeast. J Cell Biol 1999; 144:83-98.
33. Cai L, Makhov AM, Bear JE. F-actin binding is essential for coronin 1B function in vivo. J Cell Sci 2007; 120:1779-1790.
34. Gatfield J, Pieters J. Essential role for cholesterol in entry of mycobacteria into macrophages. Science 2000; 288:1647-1650.

35. Machesky LM, Reeves E, Wientjes F et al. Mammalian actin-related protein 2/3 complex localises to regions of lamellipodial protrusion and is composed of evolutionarily conserved proteins. Biochem J 1997; 328:105-112.
36. Humphries CL, Balcer HI, D'Agostino JL et al. Direct regulation of Arp2/3 complex activity and function by the actin binding protein coronin. J Cell Biol 2002; 159:993-1004.
37. Rodal AA, Sokolova O, Robins DB et al. Conformational changes in the Arp2/3 complex leading to actin nucleation. Nat Struct Mol Biol 2005; 12:26-31.
38. Föger N, Rangell L, Danilenko DM et al. Requirement for coronin 1 in T-lymphocyte trafficking and cellular homeostasis. Science 2006; 313:839-842.
39. Cai L, Marshall TW, Uetrecht AC et al. Coronin 1B coordinates Arp2/3 complex and cofilin activities at the leading edge. Cell 2007; 128:915-929.
40. Rappleye CA, Paredez AR, Smith CW et al. The coronin-like protein POD-1 is required for anterior-posterior axis formation and cellular architecture in the nematode Caenorhabditis elegans. Genes Dev 1999; 13:1838-1851.
41. Rothenberg ME, Rogers SL, Vale RD et al. Drosophila pod-1 crosslinks both actin and microtubules and controls the targeting of axons. Neuron 2003; 39:779-791.
42. Gloss A, Rivero F, Khaire N et al. Villidin, a novel WD-repeat and villin-related protein from Dictyostelium, is associated with membranes and the cytoskeleton. Mol Biol Cell 2003; 14:2716-2727.
43. Rybakin V, Gounko NV, Spate K et al. Crn7 interacts with AP-1 and is required for the maintenance of Golgi morphology and protein export from the Golgi. J Biol Chem 2006; 281:31070-31078.
44. Rybakin V, Rastetter RH, Stumpf M et al. Targeting of Crn7 to Golgi membranes requires the integrity of AP-1 complex, Src activity and presence of biosynthetic cargo. 2007; submitted.
45. Mohri K, Vorobiev S, Fedorov AA et al. Identification of functional residues on Caenorhabditis elegans actin-interacting protein 1 (UNC-78) for disassembly of actin depolymerizing factor/cofilin-bound actin filaments. J Biol Chem 2004; 279:31697-31707.
46. Hattendorf DA, Andreeva A, Gangar A et al. Structure of the yeast polarity protein Sro7 reveals a SNARE regulatory mechanism. Nature 2007; 446:567-571.
47. Bryson K, McGuffin LJ, Marsden RL et al. Protein structure prediction servers at University College London. Nucl Acids Res 2005; 33:W36-W38.
48. Mohri K, Vorobiev S, Fedorov AA et al. Identification of functional residues on Caenorhabditis elegans actin-interacting protein 1 (UNC-78) for disassembly of actin depolymerising factor/cofilin-bound actin filaments. J Biol Chem 2004; 279:31697-31707.

CHAPTER 6

Coronin:
The Double-Edged Sword of Actin Dynamics
Meghal Gandhi and Bruce L. Goode*

Abstract

Coronin is a conserved actin binding protein that promotes cellular processes that rely on rapid remodeling of the actin cytoskeleton, including endocytosis and cell motility. However, the exact mechanism by which coronin contributes to actin dynamics has remained elusive for many years. Here, we integrate observations from many groups and propose a unified model to explain how coronin controls actin dynamics through coordinated effects on Arp2/3 complex and cofilin. At the front end of actin networks, coronin protects new (ATP-rich) filaments from premature disassembly by cofilin and recruits Arp2/3 complex to filament sides, leading to nucleation, branching and network expansion. At the rear of networks, coronin has strikingly different activities, synergizing with cofilin to dismantle old (ADP-rich) filaments. Thus, coronin spatially targets Arp2/3 complex and cofilin to opposite ends of actin networks. The net effect of coronin's activities is acceleration of polarized actin subunit flux through filamentous arrays. This increases actin network plasticity and replenishes the actin monomer pool required for new filament growth.

Introduction

Dynamic remodeling of the actin cytoskeleton generates force and structural organization for diverse physiological processes, such as cell migration, endocytosis, cytokinesis and cell morphogenesis.[1] Optimal plasticity of cellular actin networks is achieved by maintaining actin filaments in a state of constant flux, where the subunits comprising filaments are turned over rapidly. There is a net addition of actin monomers at the available barbed ends of filaments and net loss of subunits from the pointed ends. New filament growth in cells is required for expansion of existing actin networks, construction of new actin arrays and force production, while the rapid disassembly of older filaments is necessary for sustaining network plasticity and replenishing the pool of assembly-competent actin monomers available for new growth. This dynamic flux ('turnover') of networks allows them to be reconfigured rapidly in response to spatial and temporal cues.

The growth and remodeling of actin networks in vivo is controlled with exquisite timing and precision through the concerted activities of numerous actin-associated proteins. Key points of control include filament nucleation, elongation, bundling, branching, capping and severing, in addition to monomer sequestration and recycling. Some actin-binding proteins are highly conserved across distant species and are ubiquitously expressed (e.g., cofilin, profilin, Arp2/3 complex and capping protein), thus defining a core set of actin-regulating proteins in eukaryotic cells. Other actin-binding proteins have more specific functions and tailor the properties of actin arrays to the unique requirements of each cell type or organism. While the functions of some core

*Corresponding Author: Bruce L. Goode—Department of Biology, Rosenstiel Basic Medical Science Research Center, Brandeis University, 415 South Street, Waltham, MA 02454, USA. Email: goode@brandeis.edu

The Coronin Family of Proteins, edited by Christoph S. Clemen, Ludwig Eichinger and Vasily Rybakin. ©2008 Landes Bioscience and Springer Science+Business Media.

actin-regulating proteins have been studied extensively and their biochemical and cellular functions firmly established, others have only recently begun to be characterized. One of these ubiquitous yet elusive actin-binding proteins is coronin.

In this chapter, we discuss how coronin is thought to influence actin dynamics in cells. Included below are sections describing coronin domains and physical interactions, genetic evidence supporting coronin's importance in the actin cytoskeleton, coronin regulation of Arp2/3 complex-mediated actin assembly, and coronin regulation of cofilin-mediated actin disassembly and turnover. We then integrate these functions into a unified model describing the overall effects of coronin on the dynamics of cellular actin networks.

Deconstructing Coronin: Isoforms, Domains and Interactions

Coronin was first identified in actin-myosin preparations isolated from *Dictyostelium discoideum* and was shown to bind directly to F-actin in vitro and colocalize with F-actin structures in vivo.[2] Since then, a wide variety of coronins have been characterized. Some model organisms (e.g., *Saccharomyces cerevisiae* and *Schizosaccharomyces pombe*) have a single coronin gene, while others (e.g., *Dictyostelium discoideum*, *Drosophila melanogaster* and *Caenorhabditis elegans*) have 2-3 coronin genes and mammals have up to seven different coronin-related genes.[3] Most coronins have a characteristic three-part domain layout, consisting of the β-propeller domain, followed by a highly variable 'unique' segment and a C-terminal coiled-coil domain (Fig. 1).

The β-Propeller Domain

The signature domain of coronin family proteins is the WD-repeat region.[4] Crystallization of murine Coronin 1A (lacking its coiled-coil domain) revealed that it forms a seven-bladed β-propeller structure assembled from five canonical WD repeats and two noncanonical repeats (Fig. 1).[5] In addition, two tandem stretches of conserved residues located in the C-terminal extension of the WD-repeat region closely associate with the underside of the propeller, possibly providing additional structural integrity. Although in principle β-propeller structures can support multiple protein-protein interactions, in the eighteen years that coronin has been studied only one binding partner of its propeller domain has been identified, F-actin. Binding to F-actin was first demonstrated for *Dictyostelium* coronin,[2] and later this activity was dissected for yeast coronin, where it was shown that an intact propeller domain is sufficient to bind actin filaments.[6] More recently, a single conserved actin-binding residue was identified in the mouse Coronin 1B propeller domain.[7] The next steps required to gain a deep understanding of coronin-F-actin interactions include: (1) identifying the entire actin-binding footprint on coronin, (2) defining the reciprocal coronin-binding surface(s) on F-actin and (3) determining how coronin binding might influence F-actin conformation and/or nucleotide binding state.

Unique Region

The unique region of coronin is highly variable in length and sequence and its function(s) remains poorly understood. Interestingly, the unique regions of *S. cerevisiae* Crn1 and *D. melanogaster* Dpod1 share noted sequence homology with the microtubule-binding region of mammalian MAP1B and the corresponding purified coronin proteins bind to microtubules and crosslink microtubules and actin filaments in vitro.[6,8] Genetic analyses of these two coronins are also consistent with their regulation of microtubule-based cellular functions. In yeast, low penetrance phenotypes (aberrant cytoplasmic microtubules and short cell-cycle delays) suggest that Crn1 may help promote nuclear migration.[6,9] This process involves coordinated interactions between polarized actin cables and cytoplasmic microtubules, which are required to translocate the nucleus to the mother-bud neck and orient the pre-anaphase mitotic spindle to ensure faithful segregation of chromosomes. In *Drosophila*, Dpod1 is required for proper axonal guidance. This process also depends on close physical interactions and regulatory feedback cues between microtubules and cortical actin networks, which are necessary for growth cone steering and navigation.[8]

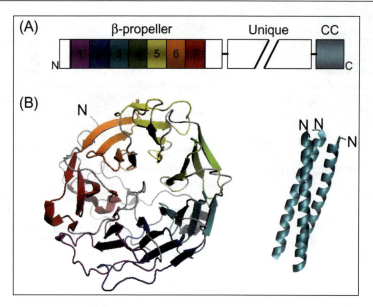

Figure 1. Coronin domain organization and protein structure. A) Schematic of coronin domain organization. The β-propeller domain is approximately 400 residues in length and comprised of seven repeats (5 WD repeats and 2 unconventional repeats; numbered and colored) flanked by short N- and C-terminal extensions (open). This is followed by the unique region (highly variable in sequence and length) and coiled-coil domain (approximately 35-50 residues in length). B) Crystal structures of mouse Coronin 1A β-propeller domain (Appleton et al 2006,[5] PDB accession number 2AQ5) and coiled-coil domain (Kammerer et al 2005,[53] PDB accession number 2AKF). The blades of the β-propeller are color-coded to match the schematic in A. The C-terminal extension (dark grey) associates with the underside of the blades. The coiled-coil domain of Coronin 1A (shown) forms parallel trimers, whereas the coiled-coil domains of some other coronins form dimers. N, amino terminus.

Coiled-Coil Domain

Remarkably, the smallest functional region of coronin, its C-terminal coiled-coil domain (~35-50 residues, 4-7 heptad repeats), mediates at least three different functional interactions (with itself, F-actin and Arp2/3 complex). The first interaction defined for the coiled-coil domain was homo-oligomerization (forming dimers or trimers), which is required for actin filament bundling by coronin (Fig. 2A).[6,10-12] This observation has led to the widely accepted model that coronin bundles actin filaments through multimerization of its β-propeller actin binding site domain (Fig. 2B). However, oligomerization has only been demonstrated in solution in the absence of F-actin and thus alternative models for bundling remain possible. For instance, bundling may result from individual (non-oligomerized) coronin molecules utilizing two separate actin-binding sites to crosslink filaments (Fig. 2C). In support of this alternative model, deletion of the coiled-coil domain dramatically weakens the actin binding affinity of coronin.[7,13] Although one study reported that the coiled-coil domain alone does not bind F-actin and suggested that the ability of the coiled-coil domain to increase actin-binding affinity is due to avidity (multimerization of the β-propeller domain),[7] other studies have detected F-actin binding activity in the coiled-coil domain.[13,14] The presence of a second actin binding site in the coiled-coil domain would allow coronin to bundle F-actin by a mechanism using two distinct actin-binding domains (one in the β-propeller, one in the coiled-coil domain). In this model, oligomers of coronin may represent an inactive molecular state, with distribution between oligomeric and non-oligomeric forms

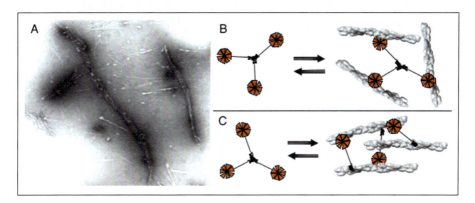

Figure 2. Actin filament bundling by coronin. A) Electron micrograph of purified actin filaments bundled by yeast coronin (Crn1). B,C) Two possible mechanisms for bundling of filaments by coronin. In the first model (B), coiled-coil mediated self-interaction of coronin multimerizes the F-actin binding β-propeller domain, thereby cross-linking filaments. In the second model (C), a single coronin polypeptide (non-oligomerized) cross-links actin filaments using two distinct actin-binding sites (in the β-propeller domain and coiled-coil domain) and coronin oligomerizes specifically when free in solution.

possibly being regulated by posttranslational modification of coronin (Fig. 2C; and see Section on Coronin-Arp2/3 Complex).

The coiled-coil domain of coronin also mediates direct interactions with the Arp2/3 complex both in vivo and in vitro.[15-17] The specific effects of coronin on Arp2/3 complex activity and how this interaction contributes to the regulation of cellular actin dynamics are addressed in Section on Coronin-Arp2/3 Complex.

What remains unclear is how these three seemingly distinct functional roles of the coiled-coil domain are integrated. Can the coiled-coil domain mediate oligomerization, F-actin binding and/or Arp2/3 complex binding simultaneously? Are there separable sites/residues in the coiled-coil domain that direct these different interactions? Answering these questions will require detailed structure-function analysis focused on the coiled-coil domain. However, regardless of the mechanism used, it is remarkable that this relatively small domain can serve as a multi-functional platform, whereas the much larger β-propeller domain has so far been implicated in binding only to F-actin.

Table 1 summarizes all of the known direct interactions and effects on actin of purified coronin proteins. From this compilation, it is apparent that F-actin binding and bundling are conserved functions of coronin. Arp2/3 complex and cofilin regulation by coronin may be equally well conserved, but this remains to be determined, as biochemical tests for these activities have been limited to a few studies so far.

Life without Coronin

All coronins examined to date (with the exception of mammalian coronin 7) bind to F-actin in vitro and localize to actin-rich cellular structures, underscoring the conservation and importance of the coronin–F-actin interaction. Genetic disruptions of coronin in *S. cerevisiae*, *D. discoideum*, *C. elegans*, *D. melanogaster*, *X. laevis* and mammals have further demonstrated the important roles coronins play in a wide variety of actin-based cellular processes (e.g., phagocytosis, endocytosis, cytokinesis, cell motility) and physiological functions (e.g., early embryonic development and lymphocyte function) (see Fig. 3).[17-22,24,26]

In *S. cerevisiae*, coronin colocalizes with F-actin at cortical sites of endocytosis.[6,9] Although a deletion of the coronin gene (*CRN1*) causes no overt phenotypes in endocytosis or actin organization, *crn1Δ* mutants exhibit specific genetic interactions with other mutations (*act1-159*, *cof1-22*

Table 1. Biochemical activities of purified coronin proteins

Species	Protein	Activities on F-actin	References
S. cerevisiae	Crn1	Binding (Kd = 5-10 nM ATP-actin) Bundling Microtubule-actin linkage Arp2/3 inhibition Regulation of cofilin-mediated actin disassembly	6,15,34,13
D. discoideum	Coronin	Binding	2
D. melanogaster	Dpod1	Bundling Microtubule-actin linkage	8
X. laevis	Xcoronin (Coronin 1C)	Binding	22
B. taurus	Coronin 1A (TACO, p57, ClipinA)	Binding Regulation of cofilin-mediated actin disassembly	47
H. sapiens	Coronin 1A (TACO, p57, ClipinA)	Binding Bundling Arp2/3 inhibition	50,51,14,25
H. sapiens	Coronin 1B	Binding (Kd = 170 nM ATP/ADP-Pi actin, Kd = 8 μM ADP-actin), Bundling Arp2/3 inhibition Regulation of cofilin-mediated actin disassembly	7,26
H. sapiens	Coronin 1C	Binding Bundling	10
H. sapiens	Coronin 2B ClipinC)	Binding	52

and arp2-21), demonstrating the importance of coronin in regulating the actin cytoskeleton.[6] Further, *CRN1* overexpression is lethal in yeast cells and causes the formation of aberrant actin loops, which can be suppressed by specific alleles of Arp2/3 complex.[6,15] In *Dictyostelium*, coronin localizes to crown-like cortical projections of cells and deletion of the coronin gene causes approximately 3-fold decreases in endocytosis and cell motility, defects in cytokinesis (which in *Dictyostelium* depends on efficient cell migration) and defects in phagocytosis.[18,19] The *C. elegans* coronin Pod-1 colocalizes with actin-rich structures found at the cell cortex and a *pod-1* gene deletion causes strong defects in anterior-posterior cell polarity and embryonic cell division.[21] In *D. melanogaster*, coronin homozygous mutations (*coro⁻/coro⁻*) are lethal at early to late pupal stages, with about 10% escaping adults. These viable adults show severe defects in legs, wings and eyes, often accompanied by reduced F-actin staining in the affected cells.[20] In addition, the *Drosophila* coronin Dpod1 is enriched in developing axons and is required for normal axonal guidance, possibly due to its above mentioned ability to crosslink actin and microtubules.[8] In *Xenopus*, Xcoronin localizes to the actin-rich cell periphery and expression in cultured A6 *Xenopus* cells of a dominant negative construct (lacking the coiled-coil domain) causes defects in the formation of lamellipodia and cell spreading.[22]

In mammalian species, the seven different coronins have distinct expression profiles and/or subcellular localization patterns and possibly different functions (reviewed by ref. 3). Genetic analysis is available for three mammalian coronins, including hematopoietic Coronin 1A and the more ubiquitously expressed Coronin 1B and Coronin 1C. Coronin 1A localizes to the F-actin rich membrane protrusions of activated T-lymphocytes,[23] and mouse *coronin1*$^{-/-}$ lymphocytes are impaired in cell motility and fail to develop uropods (retractile structures at the rear of the cell).[17] In addition, expression of a dominant negative Coronin 1A construct in human neutrophils leads to impaired phagocytosis and reduced cell spreading and adhesion.[24,25] Coronin 1B localizes to the leading edge of fibroblasts and RNAi-mediated depletion reduces retrograde actin flow, causes thinner and more densely branched actin filament networks at the leading edge and decreases membrane ruffling and cell motility.[26] Coronin 1C localizes to lamellipodia and membrane ruffles in fibroblasts and HEK293 cells[10] and RNAi-mediated depletion causes defects in wound healing and cell migration.[54]

Collectively, these genetic observations from diverse organisms point to conserved and important roles for coronin in regulating in vivo actin dynamics. In the sections below, we explore the mechanisms underlying these cellular functions.

Coronin-Arp2/3 Complex: Conditional Inhibition and Recruitment Drive Front-End Assembly

We still have much to learn about the intricacies of how coronin controls actin assembly in cells, but solid footholds have been gained in recent years. One major advance was identifying the Arp2/3 complex as a binding partner of coronin, then determining the activities of purified coronin on Arp2/3 complex and how genetic disruption of this interaction influences in vivo actin dynamics and organization.

The Arp2/3 complex is a seven subunit complex conserved in all eukaryotes. It is composed of two actin-related protein (Arp) components, Arp2 and Arp3 and five non-Arp components, p41/ARPC1, p34/ARPC2, p21/ARPC3, p20/ARPC4 and p16/ARPC5.[27] In all eukaryotic organisms and cell types examined, the Arp2/3 complex localizes to sites of dynamic actin assembly, such as the leading edge of motile fibroblasts, the dynamic cortical projections of *Dictyostelium* cells and yeast cortical endocytic actin patches.[28-30] At these sites, Arp2/3 complex performs two apparently coupled functions, actin filament nucleation and branching.[31] Nucleation involves Arp2 and Arp3 forming a pseudo-actin dimer that seeds the polymerization of actin. Branching involves association of the Arp2/3 complex with the side of an existing (mother) actin filament and nucleation of a new (daughter) filament at a 70° angle.[32] Alone, the Arp2/3 complex has inherently weak nucleation activity, but can be activated and transformed into a strong nucleator. Activation requires direct binding of Arp2/3 complex to a nucleation-promoting factor (NPF), such as a WASp/SCAR/WAVE family protein and possibly interaction with the side of a pre-existing mother filament.[31] The potent nucleation and branching activities of Arp2/3 complex must be tightly regulated in cells. This is achieved by multiple cell signaling pathways, which converge on WASp/SCAR/WAVE proteins and other NPFs to direct spatial and temporal activation of Arp2/3 complex.

In addition to localized activation by NPFs, Arp2/3 complex is regulated through direct association with coronin. The first clue to coronin-Arp2/3 functional interactions was the observation that Coronin 1A cofractionates with Arp2/3 complex isolated from neutrophil cell lysates through multiple chromatography steps.[33] Subsequently, a direct interaction between yeast Crn1 and Arp2/3 complex was reported, which was shown to depend on the Crn1 coiled-coil domain.[15] Purified Crn1 directly inhibited the nucleation activity of WASp-stimulated Arp2/3 complex in vitro (Fig. 4A). However, inhibition occurred specifically in the absence of pre-existing actin filaments and was relieved fully by the addition of preformed filaments. In the presence of filaments, full-length Crn1, which has a high-affinity interaction with F-actin,[6] recruited Arp2/3 complex to the sides of mother filaments. These observations led to a model suggesting that coronin has two distinct effects on Arp2/3 complex. It inhibits Arp2/3 complex nucleation activity in regions of the cell where pre-existing filaments are sparse, suppressing spontaneous and/or unbranched nucleation events. On the other hand, in regions where filaments are abundant (e.g., leading edge networks), coronin recruits Arp2/3 complex to the sides of existing filaments, thereby promoting

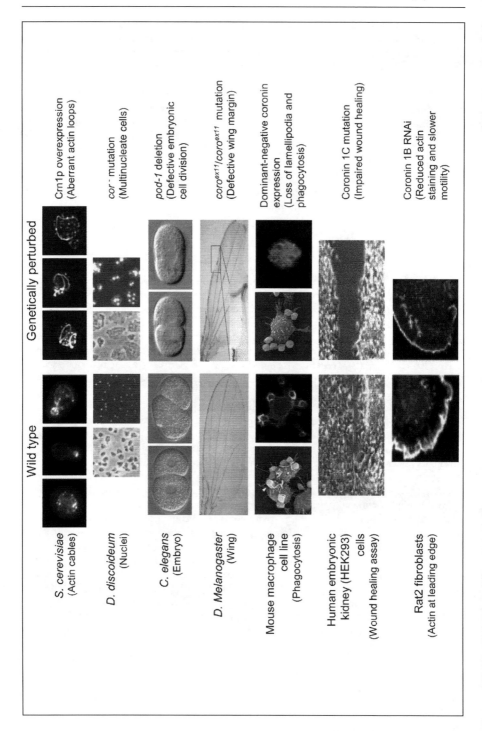

Figure 3. Legend located on opposite page.

Figure 3, opposite page. Phenotypes caused by mutation, RNAi depletion, or overexpression of coronin. Left panels are wild-type (untreated) cells or tissues. Right panels are genetically perturbed. Images were reproduced with permission from the following sources: *S. cerevisiae* and *D. discoideum* are reproduced from Humphries et al. J Cell Biol 2002; 159:993-1004 © 2002 The Rockefeller University Press and de Hostos et al. J Cell Biol 1993; 120:163-173 © 1993 The Rockefeller University Press; *C. elegans* from Rappleye et al. Genes Dev 1999; 13:2838-2851 © 1999 Cold Spring Harbor Laboratory Press; *D. melanogaster* from Bharathi et al. J Cell Sci 2004; 117:1911-1922 with permission of the Company of Biologists; Mouse macrophages from Yan et al. Mol Biol Cell 2005; 16:3077-3087; HEK293 cells and Rat2 fibroblasts are reproduced from Rosentreter et al. Exp Cell Res. 2007; 313:878-895 © 2006 and Cai et al. Cell 2007; 128:915-929 © 2007 respectively, with permission from Elsevier.

rather than inhibiting nucleation and branching (i.e., coronin reinforces the expansion of existing filament networks)[15]. By acting as a spatial regulator of Arp2/3 complex activity, coronin has a net positive effect on the assembly of Arp2/3-dependent filament networks.

The molecular mechanism for coronin inhibition of Arp2/3 complex was later addressed using electron microscopy and single particle analysis to solve the structures of free and Crn1-bound yeast Arp2/3 complexes.[34] Free Arp2/3 complex was evenly distributed among three separate conformations—'open', 'intermediate' and 'closed'. Mutational analysis and docking of the crystal structure of inactive Arp2/3 complex showed that the open conformation of the complex is inactive, whereas the closed conformation is active (primed for nucleation). Consistent with these assignments, 100% of Crn1-bound Arp2/3 complexes were in the open (inactive) conformation, whereas 100% of WASp-bound Arp2/3 complexes were in the closed (active) conformation (Fig. 4B and 4C). From these results, it was suggested that Crn1 inhibits Arp2/3 complex by stabilizing the open (inactive) conformation. These effects appear to be mediated by a direct interaction between the coronin coiled-coil domain and the p35/ARPC2 subunit of Arp2/3 complex. Three separate lines of evidence suggest this: (1) a two-hybrid interaction between the C-terminus of Crn1 and p35/ARPC2 was reported;[15] (2) electron micrographs of Crn1-bound Arp2/3 complex revealed a 40 Å diameter mass (likely to represent the β-propeller of Crn1) positioned close to p35/ARPC2;[34] (3) point mutations at a conserved solvent-exposed surface on p35/ARPC2 have been shown to abolish Crn1 interactions with Arp2/3 complex (Daugherty and Goode, unpublished data). By interacting with p35/ARPC2, coronin is in a prime position to influence Arp2/3 complex activity. The p35/ARPC2 subunit is part of the structural/functional hub of the complex, making direct contacts with three other subunits (Arp2, Arp3 and p19/ARPC4) and the sides of mother filaments. p35/ARPC2 also plays an essential role in relaying activation signals from WASP (and possibly filament side binding) to other subunits in the complex that lead to actin nucleation.[34] What remains unclear and needs to be addressed in future studies is how binding of the coronin coiled-coil domain to p35/ARPC2 affects interactions of this subunit with the sides of mother filaments and affects filament branch formation and turnover.

In vivo regulation of Arp2/3 complex by yeast coronin was suggested by two separate genetic observations. Combining *crn1Δ* and *arp2-21* mutations caused synthetic defects in cell growth and overexpression of Crn1 was lethal and led to the formation of aberrant actin loop structures decorated with Arp2/3 complex. It was suggested that these defects arise from coronin mis-regulation of Arp2/3 complex, because they are suppressed by specific alleles of p35/Arc35 or by deleting the Arp2/3-interacting coiled-coil domain of Crn1.[15]

More recently, it has been found that coronin-Arp2/3 complex interactions and inhibitory effects are conserved in mammals.[16,17,25,26] These studies have provided important new insights into how Coronin-Arp2/3 complex interactions affect the assembly of cellular actin networks and actin-based processes such as cell motility and phagocytosis. One study showed that mouse Coronin 1B coimmunoprecipitates with Arp2/3 complex and that this interaction is important for motility.[16] Further, RNAi-mediated depletion of Coronin 1B in Rat2 fibroblast cells decreased lamellipodial advancement and protrusion persistence, leading to a decrease in whole-cell motility.[26] Interestingly, the barbed end zone at the leading edge of the motile cells, which normally

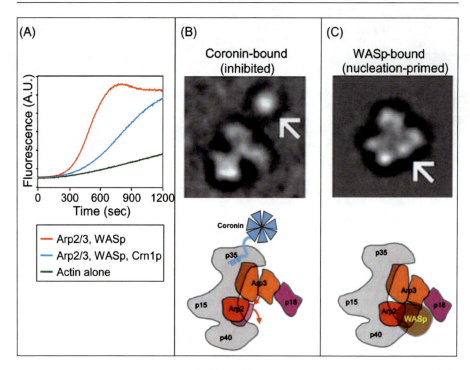

Figure 4. Regulation of Arp2/3 complex by coronin. A) Effects of purified full-length yeast coronin (Crn1) on WASp/Arp2/3 complex-induced assembly of pyrene-actin. Reactions contain 2 μM rabbit skeletal muscle actin (5% pyrene-labeled) combined with 20 nM yeast Arp2/3 complex, 20 nM GST-VCA domain of yeast WASp and/or 1 μM Crn1, as indicated. B) Top: Electron micrograph of purified yeast Arp2/3 complex bound to full-length Crn1, which stabilizes Arp2/3 complex in the 'open' (inactive) conformation. Arrow points to a new mass observed specifically in the presence of Crn1, which likely represents its β-propeller domain. Bottom: Cartoon showing coronin coiled-coil domain binding to the p35/ARPC2 subunit of Arp2/3 complex. Red arrows denote hypothesized subunit rearrangements in Arp2/3 complex that occur upon activation. C) Top: Electron micrograph of purified yeast Arp2/3 complex bound to full-length yeast WASp, which stabilizes Arp2/3 complex in the 'closed' (nucleation-primed) conformation. Arrow points to a new mass observed specifically in the presence of WASp. Bottom: Cartoon showing WASp interacting with the Arp2, Arp3 and p40 subunits. Images in B and C were reproduced from Rodal et al. Nat Struct Mol Biol 2005; 12:26-31© 2005 with permission from Macmillan Publishers Ltd.

grows very rapidly, was significantly narrowed after Coronin 1B depletion. This suggests that loss of cororin may have caused a reduction in barbed end generation at the leading edge, consistent with the model described above for spatial control of Arp2/3 complex regulation by coronin. In another study, it was suggested that mouse Coronin 1A controls steady-state F-actin levels via an Arp2/3 complex-dependent mechanism in T-lymphocytes.[17] Phalloidin staining revealed that F-actin levels are elevated in *coronin1*$^{-/-}$ T-cells. Further, expression of wild type Coronin 1A in the mutant cells restored F-actin levels back to the wild type state, but expression of Coronin 1A mutants impaired in Arp2/3 complex interactions (see below) failed to restore F-actin levels. The implication of these observations is that interactions between Coronin 1A and Arp2/3 complex are important for maintaining the F-actin equilibrium in T-cells. However, the truncation made in coronin for this study not only disrupts binding to Arp2/3 complex, but also deletes an important actin binding domain that influences cofilin activity (see below). Thus, it is equally plausible that disruption of coronin and cofilin synergy by this mutant leads to elevated steady state F-actin.

Coronin-Arp2/3 complex interactions also can be regulated by posttranslational modification. Protein kinase C (PKC) phosphorylation of Serine 2 on Coronin 1B weakens coronin-Arp2/3 complex interactions and reduces the speed of fibroblast migration in single cell tracking assays, but has no effect on Coronin 1B localization.[16] Further, a phospho-mimetic allele of Coronin 1B (S2D) shows weakened interactions with Arp2/3 complex, whereas a nonphosphorylatable Coronin 1B mutant (S2A) shows strengthened interactions with Arp2/3 complex. Coronin 1A interactions with Arp2/3 complex may also be regulated by coronin phosphorylation. This is suggested by the observation that wild type Coronin 1A reverses the elevated F-actin levels in $cororin1^{-/-}$ T-cells, while Coronin 1A (S2D, or lacking coiled-coil domain) mutants that fail to interact with Arp2/3 complex are unable to do so. It is not yet clear how a phosphorylated residue located in the coronin β-propeller domain affects Arp2/3 complex interactions that are mediated by the more distal coiled-coil domain. However, one possibility is that the β-propeller domain, when phosphorylated, binds to the coiled-coil domain to disrupt interactions with Arp2/3 complex. It also waits to be seen whether other coronins are phosphorylated at or near Serine 2 and this regulatory mechanism is conserved. There is strong evidence for coronin phosphorylation in other cell types and organisms. Two-dimensional gel analysis suggests that Coronin 1C expressed in HEK293 fibroblasts is phosphorylated.[10] In murine macrophages, the biochemical distribution of Coronin 1A between ~200 kDa and ~400-600 kDa complexes is regulated by PI-3 kinase.[35] The Golgi membrane associated fraction of human Coronin 7 expressed in NIH 3T3 fibroblasts is phosphorylated at tyrosine residues.[56] Further, yeast Crn1 is phosphorylated at multiple sites by Pho85/Cdk5 kinase (C. Humphries and B. Andrews, personal communication) and coronin and Cdk5 have been copurified with ubiquitin ligase Mib1 from neuronal postsynaptic densities.[36]

In summary, the coronin-Arp2/3 complex interaction is highly conserved across distantly related species and depends on a direct physical interaction between the coronin coiled-coil domain and a conserved surface on the p35/ARPC2 subunit of Arp2/3 complex. This interaction is regulated by coronin phosphorylation at Serine 2 in mammalian cells. Binding of coronin stabilizes the open (inactive) conformation of Arp2/3 complex, suppressing actin nucleation until these inhibitory effects are overridden by association of coronin: Arp2/3 with pre-existing filaments. Coronin actually assists in recruiting Arp2/3 complex to the sides of pre-existing filaments, thereby promoting actin nucleation and branching. Thus, coronin has the unique ability to spatially control Arp2/3 complex activity, selectively promoting the growth and expansion of existing networks. How coronin may affect actin filament branch turnover and Arp2/3 complex recycling remains to be determined.

Coronin Influence on Cofilin Activity: Protect the Front, Dismantle the Rear?

While actin nucleation represents one key control point in determining the dynamic behavior of cellular actin networks, an equally important point of control is filament disassembly. Only by maintaining actin polymers in a state of rapid turnover can cells maintain a pool of assembly-competent actin subunits for new growth and reorganize their networks rapidly in response to signals. Replenishment of subunits is accelerated by cellular factors that selectively destabilize and depolymerize the older (ADP-bound) filaments in networks. Cofilin (also called ADF) plays a central role in this process and recently it has emerged that coronin assists cofilin in driving these events.

Cofilins are a widely conserved family of proteins that accelerate actin network disassembly and are required for dynamic actin-based processes, including cell motility, endocytosis and cytokinesis.[37] Cofilin binds to the sides of actin filaments in a cooperative manner and increases the twist of filaments, leading to filament severing and disassembly. Cofilin promotes filament disassembly in concert with several other conserved actin-binding proteins, each of which makes a mechanistically distinct contribution to turnover. These include actin-interacting protein-1 (Aip1),[38-40] cyclase-associated protein (CAP),[41-44] twinfilin[45,46] and now coronin.

The first clue to the coronin-cofilin functional connection came from genetic interaction studies in yeast, where combining a *crn1Δ* mutation with a hypomorphic cofilin allele (*cof1-22*) caused synthetic defects in cell growth and actin organization.[6] Similar genetic interactions were observed between *crn1Δ* and *act1-159*, an allele of actin with decreased rates of actin turnover. More recently, it was found that *crn1Δ* causes a 4-fold reduction in rate of actin filament turnover in cells and that purified Crn1 synergizes biochemically with cofilin in severing and disassembling actin filaments.[13] This functional interaction between coronin and cofilin appears to be conserved in mammals, as Brieher et al[47] biochemically isolated mammalian Coronin 1A and Aip1 as cellular factors required (together with cofilin) to promote the rapid disassembly of *Listeria* actin tails and sustain *Listeria* motility. Together, Coronin 1A and Aip1 accelerated cofilin-mediated disassembly of tails by ~10-fold, with Coronin 1A contributing about ~3-fold to this effect. These observations also agree with an earlier report showing that coronin and cofilin are abundant components of isolated *Listeria* tails.[48]

Further in vivo evidence for coronin function in promoting F-actin disassembly comes from a study on T-lymphocytes, where Coronin 1A genetic disruption led to an increase in F-actin levels and a concomitant decrease in G-actin levels.[17] In addition, mammalian Coronin 1B has been shown to regulate cofilin activity in migrating fibroblasts by recruiting Slingshot phosphatase to the lamellipodium. Phosphorylated (inactive) cofilin is then dephosphorylated (activated) by Slingshot, leading to filament severing.[26] Accordingly, cells depleted of Coronin 1B by RNAi have higher levels of phospho-cofilin and decreased rates of retrograde actin flow and cell motility. Although Slingshot is not conserved in *S. cerevisiae* and *C. elegans*, it is possible that other phosphatases perform this function and analogously control coronin and/or cofilin activities in these organisms.

While a conserved cellular function for coronin in regulating cofilin-dependent actin disassembly is clear, the mechanism underlying these effects is only just emerging. To describe the current understanding of coronin mechanism in actin disassembly, it is beneficial to first consider the separate effects of its β-propeller and coiled-coil domains on cofilin activity and then combine this knowledge to arrive at a more complete picture of this mechanism.

Recent analyses using purified proteins have demonstrated that a fragment of yeast Crn1 that includes the β-propeller domain but lacks the coiled-coil domain biochemically synergizes with cofilin in severing and disassembling actin.[13] The same fragment of Crn1 genetically complements loss of *CRN1* in a *cof1-22* background, suggesting that the coronin-cofilin functional synergy occurs in vivo. Further, this synergy depends on direct binding of the Crn1 β—propeller to F-actin, an interaction that alters the twist of actin filaments, possibly predisposing them for cofilin binding (B. Goode and A. McGough, unpublished data). A second possibility, not mutually exclusive from the first, is that coronin more directly recruits cofilin to actin filaments. While there is no evidence available to suggest a direct physical interaction between coronin and cofilin in solution, it remains possible that they associate when bound to actin filaments.

In contrast to the stimulatory effects of the β-propeller domain of Crn1 on cofilin activity, the coiled-coil domain of Crn1 inhibits filament binding and severing by cofilin.[13] Moreover, full-length yeast and mammalian coronin proteins (which include the coiled-coil domain) inhibit filament binding and severing by coronin.[7,13] Thus, the coiled-coil domain is both required and sufficient for cofilin inhibition and the inhibitory effects of the coiled-coil domain appear to dominate over the positive synergistic effects of the β-propeller domain with cofilin. Mechanistically, the inhibitory effect of the coiled-coil domain stems from its ability to bind F-actin and competitively displace cofilin from filaments.[13] These effects may be conserved, because F-actin-binding activity has been reported for a coiled-coil domain containing fragment of mammalian Coronin 1A.[14] In addition, full-length mammalian Coronin 1B competitively displaces cofilin from F-actin and reciprocally, cofilin binding to F-actin displaces Coronin 1B from filaments.[7] Thus, not only does the coiled-coil domain function to directly regulate Arp2/3 complex, it also protects actin filaments from the effects of cofilin.

How can the observation that full-length yeast Crn1 and mammalian Coronin 1B inhibit cofilin in vitro be reconciled with genetic observations showing that both of these coronins increase (rather than decrease) rates of cofilin-mediated actin turnover in vivo? Further, how can biochemical inhibition by these two coronins be reconciled with data from Brieher et al[47] showing that Coronin 1A enhances (rather than inhibits) cofilin-mediated disassembly of *Listeria* tails? We postulate that coronin has highly distinct effects on older (ADP-bound) versus newer (ATP-bound) actin filaments. Specifically, presense of the coiled-coil domain enables cororin to bind to and selectively protect ATP-rich F-actin from cofilin, thus protecting newly assembled actin filaments at the front end of networks. In contrast, ADP-rich filaments at the rear of networks are not protected by coronin and thus are vulnerable to cofilin attack. By this mechanism, nucleotide-dependent interactions of cororin with F-actin would switch coronin's influence on cofilin from prohibitive to stimulatory. This model is supported by a recent study showing that full-length Coronin 1B binds to ATP/ADP+Pi-F-actin with 47 times greater affinity compared to ADP-F-actin.[7] It is also consistent with the ADP-F-actin binding affinity of full-length Coronin 1B (Kd = 8 μM) matching the ATP-F-actin binding affinity of a truncated Crn1 lacking the coiled-coil domain. Suggesting that the coiled-coil domain does not contribute substantially to ADP-F-actin binding.[13] Thus, filaments comprised of ADP-actin would be rapidly dismantled by the synergistic effects of the coronin β-propeller domain and cofilin. These unique abilities of coronin to act differentially on new versus old filaments would intensify the inherent binding preference of cofilin for ADP-F-actin compared to ATP-actin[55] and sharpen the contrast in polarized behavior between actin dynamics at the front and the rear of networks.

Such a model would also explain some of the observations from Brieher et al[47] that had been seemingly at odds with observations from other studies. They showed that Coronin 1A enhances (rather than inhibits) cofilin-mediated actin disassembly. We suggest that this difference is due to the substrate used for actin disassembly, *Listeria* tails, which are likely to have large regions of ADP-actin at the rear of the tails, where the coronin-cofilin synergy was observed. Further, Brieher et al[47] observed that Coronin 1A substantially (4-5 fold) increased cofilin recruitment to *Listeria* tails, but only modestly (1.5-fold) increased cofilin recruitment to purified F-actin. Again, this difference may be explained by *Listeria* tails being richer in ADP-actin compared to purified actin filaments. Consistent with this possibility, a close examination of the data in this study suggests that cofilin is recruited preferentially to one end of the *Listeria* tail (Fig. 6B in Brieher et al[47]), presumably the ADP-actin-rich trailing end.

An Integrated Working Model for Coronin Mechanism and Function

In the previous two sections, we have described how coronin regulates Arp2/3 complex-mediated actin assembly and cofilin-mediated actin disassembly. How are these apparently separate functions of coronin coordinated spatially and temporally and what is the integrated effect of these two activities on actin networks? A working model is presented in Figure 5. At the front end of the actin network, coronin binds with high affinity to the ATP/ADP+Pi-rich actin filaments using two separate actin-binding sites (in the β-propeller domain and coiled-coil domain). These interactions recruit Arp2/3 complex to the sides of filaments to promote nucleation and branching. Although coronin inhibits Arp2/3 complex activity in the absence of filaments (perhaps suppressing nucleation in cytoskeleton-free regions of the cytoplasm), it actually recruits Arp2/3 complex to preexisting filaments, where coronin inhibition is overridden and nucleation and branching proceed. A second important effect of coronin binding to ATP-F-actin at the front end of the network is protection from cofilin attack. Binding of the coiled-coil domain of coronin to F-actin blocks the ability of cofilin to bind and sever ATP-actin filaments. Thus, the net effect of coronin activities at the leading edge is protection of newly formed actin filaments from cofilin and enhancement of Arp2/3 complex-mediated assembly and expansion of branched networks.

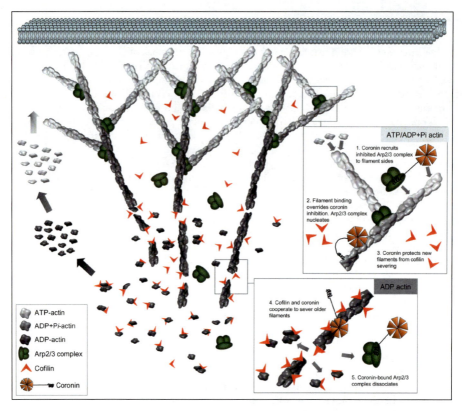

Figure 5. Model for coronin regulation of actin dynamics. This model applies to actin networks in a wide range of species and cell types (e.g., actin arrays found at the leading edge of migrating vertebrate cells and endocytic actin patches in yeast). New filament growth occurs close to the plasma membrane, producing filaments enriched in ATP-actin and ADP+Pi-actin. Older filaments comprised of ADP-actin arise after nucleotide hydrolysis and Pi release and are found at the rear of networks, distal to the cell cortex. In the cytosol where filament levels are relatively low, coronin inhibits Arp2/3 complex activity. However, at the cortex where filament levels are high, coronin inhibition is overridden. Coronin has high affinity for ATP-actin but not ADP-actin (Cai et al 2007[7]) and helps recruit Arp2/3 complex to the sides of ATP-actin filaments (Humphries et al 2002[15]). This promotes nucleation and branching at the front of networks. Two distinct actin-binding sites in coronin (β-propeller and coiled-coil domains) contribute to binding ATP-actin filaments. The interaction of coronin's coiled-coil domain with ATP-actin competitively protects filaments from cofilin binding and severing, thus preventing premature fragmentation and disassembly of new filaments. In contrast, at the rear of networks, coronin fails to protect ADP-actin filaments and instead synergizes with cofilin in severing and depolymerizing filaments (Gandhi and Goode, submitted[13]). Thus, coronin promotes filament growth at the front of networks and filament disassembly at the rear. These activities of coronin accelerate polarized actin subunit flux through the filament arrays.

In this model, the effects of coronin at the rear of the actin network are strikingly different. Filaments are rich in ADP-actin, which dramatically weakens coronin binding to F-actin. The coiled-coil domain no longer inhibits cofilin attack, allowing the β-propeller to recruit cofilin to F-actin and synergize with cofilin in severing and depolymerizing filaments. In this manner, coronin and cofilin selectively target older ADP-rich actin filaments for demolition and thereby promote a high rate of polarized actin network turnover. As filaments are being disassembled, Arp2/3 complex and coronin dissociate and then diffuse to the front end of the network where they are employed for new rounds of actin assembly and branching. This model is consistent with the treadmilling model for branched actin arrays, where Arp2/3 complex-dependent nucleation occurs at the front of the lamellipodia and cofilin-dependent depolymerization of filaments occurs at the rear.[49]

For simplicity, we have not included in the model how the changing phosphorylation states of coronin and cofilin influence the mechanism. However, the studies of Bear and coworkers show convincingly that coronin interactions with Arp2/3 complex are governed by phosphorylation and that coronin recruitment of Slingshot phosphatase leads to cofilin-mediated F-actin disassembly.[16,26] Thus, it will be intriguing to define the precise timing and order of coronin and cofilin phosphorylation and dephosphorylation events and how they relate to the inherent differential affinity and biochemical effects of coronin and cofilin on new versus old actin filaments.

Conclusions and Perspective

In a cellular milieu of actin-binding proteins, where each makes a highly specific contribution to actin dynamics, coronin is somewhat unique in its ability to influence two separate and crucial control points, actin assembly and disassembly. These seemingly distinct aspects of actin regulation are actually tightly interwoven. While actin polymerization provides the force and directionality for many cellular processes (e.g., endocytosis, cytokinesis and cell motility), actin disassembly is required to an equal extent for replenishing the pool of monomers used for new rounds of filament assembly and allowing responsive and dynamic reorganization of networks. Coronin has properties that allow it to coordinate events in both actin assembly and disassembly.

We have integrated the observations from many groups and proposed a unified model to explain how coronin might regulate actin dynamics in a wide variety of organisms and cell types. This model suggests that coronin controls activities of the Arp2/3 complex and cofilin, spatially directing them to opposite ends of filament networks. This would have an overall effect of driving polar flux of actin subunits through filamentous networks, thereby increasing actin dynamics, consistent with genetic and biochemical analyses of many different coronins. Importantly, this is only one of many possible models, and still requires rigorous experimental testing. While it is appealing to suggest that coronins from diverse organisms share a common mechanism for controlling actin dynamics, it is also possible that their mechanisms and functions have diverged. Resolving this issue will require new biochemical studies on coronins from different species and characterization of their in vivo binding partners and functional cofactors.

There are also many other open questions and unresolved mysteries surrounding coronin function that require future attention. It is uncertain if or how coronins that lack a coiled-coil domain (e.g., Pod-1) affect cytoskeletal dynamics and/or organization, as there are only limited reports on their biochemical and cellular activities. Microtubule functions suggested for some coronins also remain poorly defined and it is unclear how interactions with microtubules and actin are coordinated. In addition, we have only a limited view of how coronin is regulated by phosphorylation. Recently, important breakthroughs were made on this front illustrating how phosphorylation of coronin can affect its interactions with Arp2/3 complex. This likely represents only the tip of the iceberg on coronin phospho-regulation and thus more intense future investigations are needed to define coronin post-translational modifications and effects. Last, there is the question of how diverse mammalian coronin isoforms are targeted to different subcellular locations (e.g., lamellipodia, stress fibers and Golgi) and whether they have distinct roles in controlling different actin structures at these locations.

Acknowledgements

We are indebted to Melissa Chesarone, Karen Daugherty, Eugeno de Hostos, Amy Grace DuPage, Avital Rodal and Elsie Yu for comments on the chapter and valuable discussions. This work was supported in part by a grant from the NIH to B.G. (GM063691). Owing to space restrictions, we were unable to include all published works on coronin and we apologize to the authors of papers omitted.

References

1. Pollard TD, Borisy GG. Cellular motility driven by assembly and disassembly of actin filaments. Cell 2003; 112(4):453-465.
2. de Hostos EL, Bradtke B, Lottspeich F et al. Coronin, an actin binding protein of Dictyostelium discoideum localized to cell surface projections, has sequence similarities to G protein beta subunits. EMBO J 1991; 10(13):4097-4104.
3. Uetrecht AC, Bear JE. Coronins: the return of the crown. Trends Cell Biol 2006; 16(8):421-426.
4. de Hostos EL. The coronin family of actin-associated proteins. Trends Cell Biol 1999; 9(9):345-350.
5. Appleton BA, Wu P, Wiesmann C. The crystal structure of murine coronin-1: a regulator of actin cytoskeletal dynamics in lymphocytes. Structure 2006; 14(1):87-96.
6. Goode BL, Wong JJ, Butty AC et al. Coronin promotes the rapid assembly and cross-linking of actin filaments and may link the actin and microtubule cytoskeletons in yeast. J Cell Biol 1999; 144(1):83-98.
7. Cai L, Makhov AM, Bear JE. F-actin binding is essential for coronin 1B function in vivo. J Cell Sci 2007; 120(Pt 10):1779-1790.
8. Rothenberg ME, Rogers SL, Vale RD et al. Drosophila pod-1 crosslinks both actin and microtubules and controls the targeting of axons. Neuron 2003; 39(5):779-791.
9. Heil-Chapdelaine RA, Tran NK, Cooper JA. The role of Saccharomyces cerevisiae coronin in the actin and microtubule cytoskeletons. Curr Biol 1998; 8(23):1281-1284.
10. Spoerl Z, Stumpf M, Noegel AA et al. Oligomerization, F-actin interaction and membrane association of the ubiquitous mammalian coronin 3 are mediated by its carboxyl terminus. J Biol Chem 2002; 277(50):48858-48867.
11. Oku T, Itoh S, Ishii R et al. Homotypic dimerization of the actin-binding protein p57/coronin-1 mediated by a leucine zipper motif in the C-terminal region. Biochem J 2005; 387(Pt 2):325-331.
12. Gatfield J, Albrecht I, Zanolari B et al. Association of the leukocyte plasma membrane with the actin cytoskeleton through coiled coil-mediated trimeric coronin 1 molecules. Mol Biol Cell 2005; 16(6):2786-2798.
13. Gandhi M, Goode BL. Coronin promotes in vivo turnover of actin networks by nucleotide-sensitive regulation of cofilin effects on F-actin. submitted.
14. Liu CZ, Chen Y, Sui SF. The identification of a new actin-binding region in p57. Cell Res 2006; 16(1):106-112.
15. Humphries CL, Balcer HI, D'Agostino JL et al. Direct regulation of Arp2/3 complex activity and function by the actin binding protein coronin. J Cell Biol 23 2002; 159(6):993-1004.
16. Cai L, Holoweckyj N, Schaller MD et al. Phosphorylation of coronin 1B by protein kinase C regulates interaction with Arp2/3 and cell motility. J Biol Chem 2005; 280(36):31913-31923.
17. Foger N, Rangell L, Danilenko DM et al. Requirement for coronin 1 in T-lymphocyte trafficking and cellular homeostasis. Science 2006; 313(5788):839-842.
18. de Hostos EL, Rehfuess C, Bradtke B et al. Dictyostelium mutants lacking the cytoskeletal protein coronin are defective in cytokinesis and cell motility. J Cell Biol 1993; 120(1):163-173.
19. Maniak M, Rauchenberger R, Albrecht R et al. Coronin involved in phagocytosis: dynamics of particle-induced relocalization visualized by a green fluorescent protein Tag. Cell 1995; 83(6):915-924.
20. Bharathi V, Pallavi SK, Bajpai R et al. Genetic characterization of the Drosophila homologue of coronin. J Cell Sci 2004; 117(Pt 10):1911-1922.
21. Rappleye CA, Paredez AR, Smith CW et al. The coronin-like protein POD-1 is required for anterior-posterior axis formation and cellular architecture in the nematode caenorhabditis elegans. Genes Dev 1999; 13(21):2838-2851.
22. Mishima M, Nishida E. Coronin localizes to leading edges and is involved in cell spreading and lamellipodium extension in vertebrate cells. J Cell Sci 1999; 112 (Pt 17):2833-2842.
23. Nal B, Carroll P, Mohr E et al. Coronin-1 expression in T-lymphocytes: insights into protein function during T-cell development and activation. Int Immunol 2004; 16(2):231-240.
24. Yan M, Collins RF, Grinstein S et al. Coronin-1 function is required for phagosome formation. Mol Biol Cell 2005; 16(7):3077-3087.
25. Yan M, Di Ciano-Oliveira C, Grinstein S et al. Coronin function is required for chemotaxis and phagocytosis in human neutrophils. J Immunol 2007; 178(9):5769-5778.
26. Cai L, Marshall TW, Uetrecht AC et al. Coronin 1B coordinates Arp2/3 complex and cofilin activities at the leading edge. Cell 2007; 128(5):915-929.
27. Machesky LM, Gould KL. The Arp2/3 complex: a multifunctional actin organizer. Curr Opin Cell Biol 1999; 11(1):117-121.
28. Welch MD, DePace AH, Verma S et al. The human Arp2/3 complex is composed of evolutionarily conserved subunits and is localized to cellular regions of dynamic actin filament assembly. J Cell Biol 1997; 138(2):375-384.

29. Winter D, Podtelejnikov AV, Mann M et al. The complex containing actin-related proteins Arp2 and Arp3 is required for the motility and integrity of yeast actin patches. Curr Biol 1997; 7(7):519-529.
30. Insall R, Muller-Taubenberger A, Machesky L et al. Dynamics of the Dictyostelium Arp2/3 complex in endocytosis, cytokinesis and chemotaxis. Cell Motil Cytoskeleton 2001; 50(3):115-128.
31. Goley ED, Welch MD. The ARP2/3 complex: an actin nucleator comes of age. Nat Rev Mol Cell Biol 2006; 7(10):713-726.
32. Mullins RD, Heuser JA, Pollard TD. The interaction of Arp2/3 complex with actin: nucleation, high affinity pointed end capping and formation of branching networks of filaments. Proc Natl Acad Sci USA 1998; 95(11):6181-6186.
33. Machesky LM, Reeves E, Wientjes F et al. Mammalian actin-related protein 2/3 complex localizes to regions of lamellipodial protrusion and is composed of evolutionarily conserved proteins. Biochem J 1997; 328 (Pt 1):105-112.
34. Rodal AA, Sokolova O, Robins DB et al. Conformational changes in the Arp2/3 complex leading to actin nucleation. Nat Struct Mol Biol 2005; 12(1):26-31.
35. Didichenko SA, Segal AW, Thelen M. Evidence for a pool of coronin in mammalian cells that is sensitive to PI 3-kinase. FEBS Lett 2000; 485(2-3):147-152.
36. Choe EA, Liao L, Zhou JY et al. Neuronal morphogenesis is regulated by the interplay between cyclin-dependent kinase 5 and the ubiquitin ligase mind bomb 1. J Neurosci 2007; 27(35):9503-9512.
37. Bamburg JR. Proteins of the ADF/cofilin family: essential regulators of actin dynamics. Annu Rev Cell Dev Biol 1999; 15:185-230.
38. Aizawa H, Katadae M, Maruya M et al. Hyperosmotic stress-induced reorganization of actin bundles in Dictyostelium cells over-expressing cofilin. Genes Cells 1999; 4(6):311-324.
39. Okada K, Obinata T, Abe H. XAIP1: a Xenopus homologue of yeast actin interacting protein 1 (AIP1), which induces disassembly of actin filaments cooperatively with ADF/cofilin family proteins. J Cell Sci 1999; 112 (Pt 10):1553-1565.
40. Rodal AA, Tetreault JW, Lappalainen P et al. Aip1p interacts with cofilin to disassemble actin filaments. J Cell Biol 1999; 145(6):1251-1264.
41. Moriyama K, Yahara I. Human CAP1 is a key factor in the recycling of cofilin and actin for rapid actin turnover. J Cell Sci 2002; 115(Pt 8):1591-1601.
42. Balcer HI, Goodman AL, Rodal AA et al. Coordinated regulation of actin filament turnover by a high-molecular-weight Srv2/CAP complex, cofilin, profilin and Aip1. Curr Biol 2003; 13(24):2159-2169.
43. Bertling E, Hotulainen P, Mattila PK et al. Cyclase-associated protein 1 (CAP1) promotes cofilin-induced actin dynamics in mammalian nonmuscle cells. Mol Biol Cell 2004; 15(5):2324-2334.
44. Mattila PK, Quintero-Monzon O, Kugler J et al. A high-affinity interaction with ADP-actin monomers underlies the mechanism and in vivo function of Srv2/cyclase-associated protein. Mol Biol Cell 2004; 15(11):5158-5171.
45. Goode BL, Drubin DG, Lappalainen P. Regulation of the cortical actin cytoskeleton in budding yeast by twinfilin, a ubiquitous actin monomer-sequestering protein. J Cell Biol 1998; 142(3):723-733.
46. Moseley JB, Okada K, Balcer HI et al. Twinfilin is an actin-filament-severing protein and promotes rapid turnover of actin structures in vivo. J Cell Sci 2006; 119(Pt 8):1547-1557.
47. Brieher WM, Kueh HY, Ballif BA et al. Rapid actin monomer-insensitive depolymerization of Listeria actin comet tails by cofilin, coronin and Aip1. J Cell Biol 2006; 175(2):315-324.
48. David V, Gouin E, Troys MV et al. Identification of cofilin, coronin, Rac and capZ in actin tails using a Listeria affinity approach. J Cell Sci 1998; 111 (Pt 19):2877-2884.
49. Svitkina TM, Borisy GG. Arp2/3 complex and actin depolymerizing factor/cofilin in dendritic organization and treadmilling of actin filament array in lamellipodia. J Cell Biol 1999; 145(5):1009-1026.
50. Suzuki K, Nishihata J, Arai Y et al. Molecular cloning of a novel actin-binding protein, p57, with a WD repeat and a leucine zipper motif. FEBS Lett 1995; 364(3):283-288.
51. Oku T, Itoh S, Okano M et al. Two regions responsible for the actin binding of p57, a mammalian coronin family actin-binding protein. Biol Pharm Bull 2003; 26(4):409-416.
52. Nakamura T, Takeuchi K, Muraoka S et al. A neurally enriched coronin-like protein, ClipinC, is a novel candidate for an actin cytoskeleton-cortical membrane-linking protein. J Biol Chem 1999; 274(19):13322-13327.
53. Kammerer RA, Kostrewa D, Progias P et al. A conserved trimerization motif controls the topology of short coiled coils. Proc Natl Acad Sci USA 2005; 102(39):13891-13896.
54. Rosentreter A, Hofmann A, Xavier CP et al. Coronin 3 involvement in F-actin-dependent processes at the cell cortex. Exp Cell Res 2007; 313(5):878-895.
55. Blanchoin L, Pollard TD. Mechanism of interaction of Acanthamoeba actophorin (ADF/Cofilin) with actin filaments. J Biol Chem 1999; 274(22):15538-15546.
56. Rybakin V, Stumpf M, Schulze A et al. Coronin 7, the mammalian POD-1 homologue, localizes to the Golgi apparatus. FEBS Lett 2004; 573(1-3):161-167.

CHAPTER 7

Invertebrate Coronins

Maria C. Shina and Angelika A. Noegel*

Abstract

Coronins are highly conserved among species, but their function is far from being understood in detail. Here we will introduce members of the family of coronin like proteins from *Drosophila melanogaster*, *Caenorhabditis elegans* and the social amoeba *Dictyostelium discoideum*. Genetic data from *D. discoideum* and *D. melanogaster* revealed that coronins in general are important regulators of many actin-dependent processes.

Coronins, a Versatile Family

The actin cytoskeleton is important for cell morphology and cell motility and its polymerization state can change rapidly in response to a variety of signals. Cytoskeletal dynamics are an essential component of many physiological processes, such as trafficking of intracellular vesicles, cell motility or the migration of cells during immune responses and tissue morphogenesis.[1] They are regulated by various actin-binding proteins. Coronins form one of the many groups of actin cytoskeleton regulators. Coronin was identified in the social amoeba *D. discoideum*.[2] It was first observed as a major copurifying protein in a preparation of contracted actomyosin from *D. discoideum* and was proposed to be an important regulator of the actin cytoskeleton. In order to understand the cellular and biochemical function of coronins, it is important to first consider their general molecular structure. A structural characteristic of coronins is the presence of several WD40-repeats, which in other proteins, such as the β-subunit of G-proteins, form β-propeller structures and mediate protein-protein interactions.[3] Recent structural analysis revealed a seven bladed propeller for each WD40 domain in coronin and an overall fold for the WD40-repeat domain as in G-proteins.[4,5]

Most eukaryotes express two kinds of coronins referred to as short and long coronins. Short coronins have the above described structure, the long form of coronins contains two complete copies of the basic coronin motif but lacks a coiled coil C-terminal domain that is only present in short coronins and is essential for their oligomerization.[6] The functional significance of the second copy of the WD40-repeat domain is unknown. Several coronin like proteins have been identified in different invertebrate model organisms, *D. discoideum*, *D. melanogaster* and *C. elegans*. In this review we will summarize the data obtained from these organisms emphasising the results obtained from mutant analysis.

The Coronins of *D. Discoideum*

D. discoideum is a soil living amoeba frequently used as a model organism in cell and developmental biology. The amoeba shares many physiological functions with mammalian cells and is amenable to genetic manipulation.[7] Proteome-based phylogeny shows that the amoebozoa deviated from the animal-fungal lineage after the plant-animal split, but *D. discoideum* seems to have retained more of the diversity of the ancestral genome than do plants, animals or fungi (Fig. 1).[8] The

*Corresponding Author: Angelika A. Noegel—Center for Biochemistry, Medical Faculty, University of Cologne Joseph-Stelzmann-Str. 52, 50931 Cologne, Germany. Email: noegel@uni-koeln.de

The Coronin Family of Proteins, edited by Christoph S. Clemen, Ludwig Eichinger and Vasily Rybakin. ©2008 Landes Bioscience and Springer Science+Business Media.

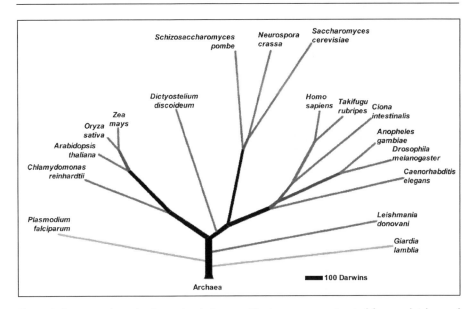

Figure 1. Proteome based eukaryotic phylogeny. The tree was constructed from a database of 5.279 orthologous protein clusters drawn from the proteomes of 17 eukaryotes shown and was rooted on 159 protein clusters that had representatives from six archaebacterial proteoms. The relative lengths of the branches are given as Darwins (where 1 Darwin = 1/2,000 of the divergence between *S. cerevisae* and humans). The figure was modified from Eichinger et al.[8]

complete protein repertoire of *D. discoideum* provides a new perspective for studying its cellular and developmental biology. At a systems level, *D. discoideum* provides a level of complexity that is greater than that of yeast, but much simpler than that of plants or animals.[9]

In *D. discoideum* three coronin like proteins have been identified, two, Coronin 7 (corB) and villidin, belonging to the class of long coronins and one, coronin or corA, the classical coronin, belonging to the short coronins (Fig. 2; Shina MC, Noegel AA unpublished). The *crn7* and the *coronin* gene are located on chromosome 1, the villidin gene *vilA* is on chromosome 5. Crn7 and coronin conform to the typical coronin structures with two and one highly conserved WD40-repeat domains (Fig. 2; Shina MC, Noegel AA unpublished), respectively, whereas villidin has a fairly unique domain structure consisting of one WD40-repeat domain followed by a gelsolin domain and a head piece (see below).

The Coronin Prototype Controls Actin Dynamics

Coronin localizes to actin rich crown-like structures on the dorsal surface of the cells, to leading edges of locomoting cells, pseudopodia, eupodia and endocytic cortical structures.[10] Detailed analysis using GFP-tagged coronin indicated its dynamic behaviour in motile cells where it continuously shuttled between the cytoplasm and front regions and accumulated in fronts that formed in response to the chemoattractant cyclic AMP (cAMP) paralleling the accumulation of F-actin.[12] Further dissection of the cAMP response revealed however that at the time of coronin recruitment at the cell cortex F-actin starts to disassemble.[11] It was therefore concluded that coronin converts the cellular response from actin polymerization to depolymerization. Rosentreter et al reported a similar differential F-actin and coronin-1C accumulation during the formation of cellular protrusions in mammalian cells.[12,13]

The involvement of coronin in various actin-driven processes has been also supported by genetic studies. In coronin-null mutants cell motility is reduced to less than half the rate in respect to wild type, cytokinesis is impaired and the rate of pino- and phagocytosis is reduced.[14,15] A more detailed

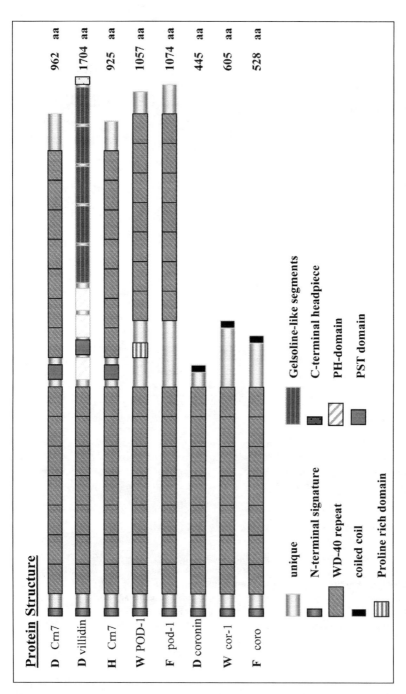

Figure 2. Comparison of domain structures of representative invertebrate coronins. From the left side, abbreviations indicating organisms, protein names, domain structures and amino acid numbers for each protein are given. All coronin proteins visualized in this figure have also been included into the comprehensive and meticulous phylogeny tree of coronins presented in chapter 4. D, *Dictyostelium discoideum*; H, *Homo sapiens*; W, *Caenorhabditis elegans*; F, *Drosophila melanogaster* (Shina MC, Noegel AA unpublished).

analysis of particle and fluid uptake revealed an intimate involvement of coronin in this process. All particle and fluid containing vacuoles are transiently surrounded by a cytoskeletal coat and by coronin. GFP-tagged coronin labeled postlysosomal vacuoles together with filamentous actin.[16-18] This association of coronin and actin at postlysosomal vacuoles emerged to be important not only for endocytosis but also for exocytosis. To show the importance of coronin and actin colocalization at postlysosomal vacuoles, cells were treated with cytochalasin. The depolymerization of actin inhibited the exocytosis rate significantly suggesting that the actin coat facilitates association of the late vacuole with the cell cortex.[17,18]

Filamentous actin is also essential for phagocytosis since cytochalasin blocks phagocytosis almost completely. Actin normally distributes along the phagocytic cup after particle attachment, while coronin accumulates at the phagocytic cup within 45 sec after attachment of a particle and separates from the phagosome within 1 min after ingestion is completed. The temporal pattern of coronin association was also seen by proteom analysis.[19,20] The role of coronin in phagocytosis is supported by mutant analysis as in coronin null mutants the phagocytosis rate is reduced by about 70%. Furthermore microscopic examination of coronin null cells showed an unusual appearance. They were mostly irregularly shaped with enlarged cell size. However, the *coronin*⁻ mutants also show that coronin is neither essential for actin assembly nor for the normal localization of the actin filaments. Moreover, the formation of cell-surface extensions called crowns and multicellular development were also observed in the absence of coronin. Although aggregation-competent cells lacking coronin moved more slowly than control cells they were still capable of chemotactic orientation in a cAMP gradient. The chemotactic responsiveness in the absence of coronin is notable because of the sequence relationship of coronin to β-subunits of G-proteins. Because of this relationship a function for coronin in regulating the transmission of signals from chemo-attractant receptors via G-proteins to the actin cytoskeleton has been suggested.[2]

When *D. discoideum* wild type cells grow and divide on bacteria, they give rise almost exclusively to mononucleated cells. During axenic growth a portion of cells containing several nuclei is found, indicating that karyokinesis is not always connected with cytokinesis under these conditions. The lack of coronin markedly enhances this tendency. This effect was interpreted in terms of the accumulation of coronin in the distal portions of dividing cells as the protein has been mainly found in polar regions of dividing cells and only some coronin was present in the cortical layer of the ingressing cleavage furrow.[21] By contrast, Fukui et al reported a coronin accumulation in the progressing cleavage furrow.[22]

The inability of *coronin*⁻ cells to divide properly under axenic conditions points to a role of coronin in cell division and illustrates that various, probably independent, actin-based mechanisms are involved in guaranteeing proper cytokinesis. In conclusion, the defects in cell growth, locomotion and cytokinesis show that coronin is involved in more than a single function of the actin system and suggest that the protein plays a general role in the reorganization of the actin cytoskeleton.[14]

In recent years *D. discoideum* has also been used as a host for infection with pathogens like *Pseudomonas aeruginosa*, *Mycobacterium avium*, *Mycobacterium marinum*, *Cryptococcus neoformans* and *Legionella pneumophila* and various *Dictyostelium* mutants have been studied with regard to uptake of bacteria and intracellular growth.[23] The *coronin* mutant proved to be susceptible to infection with *L. pneumophila* and supported intracellular growth of the bacteria better than wild type.[24,25] These results are in contrast to those obtained from macrophages where a coat formed by coronin 1A prevents the maturation of phagosomes containing living mycobacteria into lysosomes.[26]

Coronin 7, a Long Coronin in *D. Discoideum*

Coronin 7 (DCrn7) is the second coronin like protein in *D. discoideum* and the orthologue of the human Coronin 7 (Fig. 2). *D. discoideum* DCrn7 and human Coronin 7 share high homology and both possess two WD40-core repeat structures that are separated by a PST-domain (proline, serine, threonine rich region) of unknown function.[27,28]

Predictions for the structure of DCrn7 display a double propeller structure as it was shown for the *C. elegans* Actin-Interacting-Protein-1 (AIP-1).[29] Analysis of DCrn7-GFP fusions and immunofluorescence studies with specific monoclonal antibodies show a localization to actin rich structures in the cells and dot like staining in the cytosol. This contrasts with the location described for the mammalian protein which was primarily found on the Golgi apparatus.[28,30]

The 105 kDa *D. discoideum* DCrn7 is expressed throughout development and especially prominent during the aggregation state. First data from *Dcrn7* null cells show a premature development, furthermore, growth in suspension and on agar plates is decreased, cells exhibit a strong phagocytosis increase but do not show any defect in exocytosis. Moreover *Dcrn7* null cells exhibit a reduced motility in a cAMP gradient (Shina MC, Noegel AA unpublished data). Like the conventional coronin, DCrn7 accumulates at phagocytic and pinocytic cups leading to the suggestion that DCrn7 participates in the remodelling of the cortical actin cytoskeleton. A comparison of the results from the analysis of the (short) coronin and DCrn7 mutants suggests that in some processes they may act in an antagonistic fashion.

Villidin, an Unusual Coronin in *D. Discoideum*

Villidin is a 190 kDa protein from *D. discoideum* containing a coronin like domain at its N-terminus with high homology to the C-terminal WD-domain of the long coronins, which clearly places it in the coronin family, three PH domains in the middle and five gelsolin-like segments at its C-terminus followed by a villin-like headpiece. Villidin protein and mRNA are present in low amounts during growth and early aggregation, but increase during development and reach their highest levels at the tipped mound stage. The protein is present in the cytosol as well as in cytoskeletal and membrane fractions.[31] GFP-tagged villidin exhibits a similar distribution as native villidin, including a distinct colocalization with Golgi structures and ER membranes. GFP fusions of the C-terminus are uniformly dispersed in the cytoplasm whereas GFP fusions of the N-terminal WD40-repeats codistribute with F-actin and are associated with the Triton-insoluble cytoskeleton.[31] This suggests that villidin harbours the F-actin binding site in the N-terminal domain whereas the C-terminal headpiece turned out to be inactive in in vitro F-actin binding assays. The headpiece domain is present in many F-actin binding proteins and has been associated with F-actin interaction. Molecular modeling showed that the surface of the villidin headpiece did not harbor the residues that were identified as being essential for an F-actin interaction.[32]

Strains lacking villidin grow normally and can develop into fruiting bodies. Although development is not impaired, cell motility is reduced during aggregation and phototaxis during the slug stage is affected.[31] Interestingly, 55 genes are supposed to be involved in slug behavior and several of the encoded proteins regulate signal transduction pathways involving the intracellular messengers cAMP, cGMP, IP3 and Ca^{2+}.[33,34] Phototactic migration depends on the motility of individual cells that require the efficient functioning of their cytoskeleton. It was concluded that villidin plays a role in motility related processes leading to phototactic movement.

D. Melanogaster Coronins Add New Roles

The knowledge of the genome of *D. melanogaster* offers the ultimate opportunity to clarify processes ranging from the development of an organism to its behavior. During the last century, more than 1300 genes, mostly based on mutant phenotypes, were genetically identified. Interestingly, many of them were found to have counterparts in other metazoans including humans. Among the genetically identified genes, coronin or *coro* codes for the *D. melanogaster* orthologue of *D. discoideum* short coronin. At the protein sequence level coro is showing a considerable identity to a number of coronin like proteins from different organisms across the whole eukaryotic spectrum from yeast to human. Closest orthologues are coronins from mosquito (74% identity across 376 residues) and zebrafish (55% identity across 265 residues), followed by human, *Xenopus*, mouse and rat (around 54% identity across 265 residues). The protein possesses a WD40 domain, which can form a β-propeller-like structure and a C-terminal end containing a coiled-coil domain, which is implicated in dimerization at the cell periphery.[6,35] *Coro* transcripts are seen at very high levels in

0-5-hour embryos, but expression is drastically reduced after 15-20-hours and maintains a steady state level until pupal stage. Interestingly, *Enabled* (another actin binding protein) and *Costa* (a microtubule binding protein) show the highest correlation of expression to *coro*. Developmental stages at which these genes show higher levels of expression may be stages in which actin and microtubule structures play significant roles.[36]

Coro mutants were identified in a GAL4-enhancer trap screen for segmentally modulated expression patterns. Further deletion mutations that were generated by imprecise excision of the P-element affected adult morphogenesis and led to prominent wing and eye phenotypes and all homozygous females were sterile with severe defects in ovary development.[37] Closer inspection revealed a disruption of the actin cytoskeleton in imaginal discs and an altered wing disc morphology as it has been seen as result of suppressed Dpp signaling. Dpp (Decapentaplegic), a *D. melanogaster* TGF-beta orthologue, is normally transported from the source to the recipient cells through endocytosis and exocytosis of Dpp-containing vesicles. Overexpression of Dpp and its receptor Thickvein (*Tkv*), a type I receptor, in *coro* deficient cells leads to accumulation of Dpp in endocytic vesicles along the anterior-posterior boundary inhibiting the establishment of the morphogen gradient supporting the proposed vesicle-cytoskeleton interaction in which coro participates.[37-39]

The observed phenotypes of the *coro* mutants were also remarkably similar to phenotypes reported for *syntaxin1A* (*syx1A*) alleles.[38] Syx1A, a member of the SNARE complex, is required for membrane trafficking associated with synaptic vesicles or other small vesicles such as endosomes. Based on their observations the authors concluded that *D. melanogaster* coro protein functions with *syx1A* to mediate trafficking and fusion of F-actin coated vesicles with the membrane. It appears that coro displays the same biological functions like the *D. discoideum* coronin. In addition, the results on cloning and characterization of coro provide new insights into the role of the actin cytoskeleton in various developmental processes.

D. Melanogaster Pod-1 Links Actin and Microtubules

D. melanogaster in addition possesses a single long coronin like protein pod-1, that is expressed in the nervous system. Sequence analysis of the full-length cDNA for pod-1 showed that the predicted protein is 1074 aa long and 31% identical and 46% similar to *C. elegans* POD-1 (see below). *D. melanogaster* pod-1 contains two tandem WD40-repeats that likely mediate F-actin binding[40] but unlike other long coronins the two WD40 domains are not separated by a PST domain (Fig. 2). The *D. melanogaster* orthologue of other long coronins has been shown to crosslink actin and microtubules (MTs) in vitro. *D. melanogaster* pod-1 colocalizes extensively with newly assembled F-actin and often colocalizes with MTs. In developing neurons, pod-1 is concentrated in growing neurites, where it is particularly enriched at the tips of extending axons. The primary defect in embryos completely lacking *pod-1* is aberrant axon targeting. Furthermore, the level of pod-1 is critical, as postmitotic neuronal overexpression of pod-1 causes severe defects in axon path finding and induces dramatic changes in cell shape. Costaining for pod-1 and tubulin showed that in latrunculin treated cells, pod-1 relocalized from actin filaments to MTs whereas depolymerization of MTs had no effect on pod-1 localization suggesting that pod-1 has a high affinity for F-actin and a lower affinity for MTs or that its association with MTs may be regulated.

Embryos lacking zygotic expression had serious central nervous system (CNS) axon misguidance, which was however not accompanied by other general defects, suggesting that pod-1 is specifically important for axon guidance. Growth cone filopodia are required for steering but not for the extension of axons.[41] Analysis of the growth cone structure in the mutants showed no obvious disruption, as filopodia were still seen. From this it was concluded that pod-1 is not required for filopodia formation in axonal growth cones.[42,43] In addition, expression was variable as seen in nerves, which reached their targets even without any pod-1. This led to the proposal, that pod-1 is an actin-microtubule crosslinker that has functions in remodelling of the cytoskeleton during axon navigation and pod-1 may facilitate the flow of guidance information to cytoskeletal networks.

This finding, together with the endogenous pod-1 localization, is consistent with a role for pod-1 in the interaction of actin filaments and MTs in dynamic cellular structures.

C. Elegans POD-1 Is Essential for Cell Polarity

The genome of *C. elegans* was the first completely known genome of a multicellular organism. It codes for approximately 20,000 genes. Because the complete cell lineage of the species has been determined, *C. elegans* has proven especially useful for studying cellular differentiation. Polarization of cells and the asymmetric dissociation of components within cells are important in the development and function of many individual cell types, including epithelial and immune cells. The actin cytoskeleton has been shown to play an important role in establishing or maintaining polarity and the *C. elegans* embryo has become important for studying the developmental asymmetry establishment.[44]

Among actin regulatory proteins, POD-1 (stands for polarity osmotic defective 1) was identified as a protein required for anterior-posterior (a-p) axis formation during a biochemical screen for actin-interacting proteins.[45] POD-1 is a protein with homology to the long coronin family and contains two complete copies of the WD-40 domains and one proline-rich region between the coronin domains. Important regulators are the so-called *par* genes (*par*titioning defective) that control polarization of the one-cell embryo. POD-1 is polarized along the a-p axis of the one-cell embryo, suggesting it might provide a link between F-actin and the generation of polarity. Elimination of POD-1 protein from embryos results in a *par* phenotype, loss of a-p polarity but additionally also in physical defects like osmotic sensitivity. This sensitivity to external salt concentration is not found with other published polarity mutants. However, unlike the loss of other polarity or PAR proteins characterized to date, loss of POD-1 leads to dramatic and specific alterations in the internal and external structure of embryonic cells, including the formation of abnormal endocytic vesicles containing large, circular, granule-free structures, membrane protrusions, abnormal eggshells and the deposition of extracellular plaque material.[46] Analogous defects to those of POD-1 deficient worms have been observed in the *D. discoideum* coronin mutant, which led to the assumption that POD-1 has a role in intracellular trafficking and cytoskeletal organization.

The study of POD-1 spans two important biological fields of embryonic development and the cytoskeleton and appears to link developmental polarity with cell structure in a way not previously characterized in *C. elegans*, assuming POD-1 as an upstream effector of PAR-1 distribution. However, PAR-1 is not required for POD-1 asymmetric localization. Based on the fact that *D. discoideum* coronin and DCrn7 play important roles in endocytosis, colocalization of *C. elegans* POD-1 with cortical actin and cytoplasmic structures suggests a similar intracellular function and this is playing a major role in polarizing the *C. elegans* embryo.[47]

Another polarity gene, *pod-2*, was identified during large-scale screens for conditional embryonic lethal mutants.[46,48] In contrast to POD-1, *pod-2* comprises no WD40-repeats but is an Acetyl CoA Carboxylase, an enzyme that is involved in the fatty acid metabolism. A mutation of this gene *pod-2* causes also defects in anterior-posterior polarity in one-cell *C. elegans* embryos. Like loss of POD-1, loss of this gene function also results in embryos sensitive to their osmotic environment. *Pod-2* mutant embryos share a number of phenotypes with POD-1 mutant embryos suggesting that these two genes might function in a common pathway to polarize the *C. elegans* embryo. Other polarity phenotypes and osmotic defects associated with loss of POD-1 are also found in *pod-2*. Both proteins are found in the cytoplasm and if POD-1 functions in the same pathway as *pod-2*, then elimination of POD-1 in a *pod-2* mutant background should not enhance the polarity defect. Indeed, embryos lacking POD-1 and *pod-2* show the same loss of polarity as lacking either gene alone. Although POD-1 and *pod-2* share similar polarity and eggshell phenotypes, *pod-2* embryos do not display some of the nonpolarity defects associated with POD-1 embryos. They do not form abnormal endocytically derived compartments and do not develop hyaline zones.[46]

Interestingly, there is an orthologue of *pod-2* found in *D. discoideum*, *accA* (DDB0187917), which is also involved in fatty acid biosynthesis. If there is a link between POD-1 and *pod-2* there might also be a direct or indirect cooperation of *D. discoideum* Crn7 and *accA*. Moreover, *C. elegans*

POD-1 as well as *D. discoideum* coronin appear to be both involved in cytokinesis.[14] It is interesting that the BTB protein MEL-26, a substrate-specific adaptor of the CUL-3-based ligase, forms a complex with the coronin like protein POD-1 in *C. elegans*. It interacts with the entire second WD-domain and the linker region of POD-1 through its MATH-domain and POD-1 is required for proper localization of MEL26 to the cleavage furrow. On the other hand cortical localization of POD-1 is independent of MEL-26. This indicates that the MEL26/POD-1 complex at the cell cortex promotes efficient initiation and ingression of the cytokinesis furrow in vivo.[49]

In addition, the *C. elegans* genome comprises another orthologue of coronin cor-1, that reveals higher identity and more gene structure similarities to the short coronin of *D. discoideum* by also containing a single WD-40 domain and a coiled coil domain at the C-terminus.[40] For this gene five coronin mRNAs were identified in *C. elegans*. Cor-1 has an alternatively spliced exon and two exons containing cleavage sites different from the conventional splice sites.[50] Further analysis on this protein has not been carried out.

Summary

Taking all the different aspects together, coronins, apart of their common function in regulating the actin cytoskeleton, differ in their structure and length. Both short and long coronins in invertebrates seem to have almost the same distribution in the cell indicating that they might play roles in the same pathways. In *D. discoideum* coronins are located in the leading fronts and may be essential for polarization of the cell. This gives rise to the assumption that in loss of either one of the coronin like proteins polarity in these cells is disturbed. In the case of *C. elegans* there is good evidence for polarity defects, as *C. elegans* POD-1 deficient embryos show wrong distribution of PAR genes that are differentially distributed in the one-cell embryo. Also, the misguidance of neurons and the establishment of morphogen gradients in *D. melanogaster* may be linked to a distribution of polarity establishing proteins and even may play itself a role in linking these proteins to the actin cytoskeleton.

Remarkable progress has been made to understand the molecular and cellular function of these highly conserved proteins such as structural analysis and the recent discovery of a N-terminal area in human coronin 1B, providing the platform for the F-actin binding.[51] Questions that need to be addressed in the future are how these proteins are regulated and who are their binding partners. Structural analysis of some of these proteins may further reveal significant cues of presumable binding sites. However, much work is still remaining and has to be done to fully understand this interesting class of proteins.

Acknowledgements

This work was supported by the Deutsche Forschungsgemeinschaft (DFG) and the Fonds der Chemischen Industrie (FCI).

References

1. Uetrecht AC, Bear JE. Coronins: the return of the crown. Trends in Cell Biology; In Press, Corrected Proof.
2. de Hostos EL, Bradtke B, Lottspeich F et al. Coronin, an actin binding protein of Dictyostelium discoideum localized to cell surface projections, has sequence similarities to G protein beta subunits. EMBO J 1991; 10(13):4097-104.
3. Garcia-Higuera I, Fenoglio J, Li Y et al. Folding of proteins with WD-repeats: comparison of six members of the WD-repeat superfamily to the G protein beta subunit G protein heterodimers: new structures propel new questions. Biochemistry 1996; 35(44):13985-94.
4. Appleton BA, Wu P, Wiesmann C. The crystal structure of murine coronin-1: a regulator of actin cytoskeletal dynamics in lymphocytes. Structure 2006; 14(1):87-96.
5. Garcia-Higuera I, Gaitatzes C, Smith TF et al. Folding a WD repeat propeller. Role of highly conserved aspartic acid residues in the G protein beta subunit and Sec13. Analysis of the physical properties and molecular modeling of Sec13: A WD repeat protein involved in vesicular traffic. J Biol Chem 1998; 273(15):9041-9.
6. de Hostos EL. The coronin family of actin-associated proteins. Trends Cell Biol 1999; 9(9):345-50.

7. Williams RS, Boeckeler K, Graf R et al. Towards a molecular understanding of human diseases using Dictyostelium discoideum. Trends Mol Med 2006; 12(9):415-24.
8. Eichinger L, Pachebat JA, Glockner G et al. The genome of the social amoeba Dictyostelium discoideum. Nature 2005; 435(7038):43-57.
9. Chisholm RL, Firtel RA. Insights into morphogenesis from a simple developmental system. Nat Rev Mol Cell Biol 2004; 5(7):531-41.
10. Fukui Y, de Hostos E, Yumura S et al. Architectural dynamics of F-actin in eupodia suggests their role in invasive locomotion in Dictyostelium. Exp Cell Res 1999; 249(1):33-45.
11. Etzrodt M, Ishikawa HC, Dalous J et al. Time-resolved responses to chemoattractant, characteristic of the front and tail of Dictyostelium cells. FEBS Lett 2006; 580(28-29):6707-13.
12. Rosentreter A, Hofmann A, Xavier CP et al. Coronin 3 involvement in F-actin-dependent processes at the cell cortex. Exp Cell Res 2007; 313(5):878-95.
13. Hasse A, Rosentreter A, Spoerl Z et al. Coronin 3 and its role in murine brain morphogenesis. Eur J Neurosci 2005; 21(5):1155-68.
14. de Hostos EL, Rehfuess C, Bradtke B et al. Dictyostelium mutants lacking the cytoskeletal protein coronin are defective in cytokinesis and cell motility. J Cell Biol 1993; 120(1):163-73.
15. Gerisch G, Albrecht R, Heizer C et al. Chemoattractant-controlled accumulation of coronin at the leading edge of Dictyostelium cells monitored using a green fluorescent protein-coronin fusion protein. Curr Biol 1995; 5(11):1280-5.
16. Hacker U, Albrecht R, Maniak M. Fluid-phase uptake by macropinocytosis in Dictyostelium. J Cell Sci 1997; 110 (Pt 2):105-12.
17. Rauchenberger R, Hacker U, Murphy J et al. Coronin and vacuolin identify consecutive stages of a late, actin-coated endocytic compartment in Dictyostelium. Curr Biol 1997; 7(3):215-8.
18. Maniak M, Rauchenberger R, Albrecht R et al. Coronin involved in phagocytosis: dynamics of particle-induced relocalization visualized by a green fluorescent protein Tag. Cell 1995; 83(6):915-24.
19. Gotthardt D, Warnatz HJ, Henschel O et al. High-resolution dissection of phagosome maturation reveals distinct membrane trafficking phases. Mol Biol Cell 2002; 13(10):3508-20.
20. Gotthardt D, Blancheteau V, Bosserhoff A et al. Proteomics fingerprinting of phagosome maturation and evidence for the role of a Galpha during uptake. Mol Cell Proteomics 2006; 5(12):2228-43.
21. Bretschneider T, Jonkman J, Kohler J et al. Dynamic organization of the actin system in the motile cells of Dictyostelium. J Muscle Res Cell Motil 2002; 23(7-8):639-49.
22. Fukui Y, Inoue S. Cell division in Dictyostelium with special emphasis on actomyosin organization in cytokinesis. Cell Motil Cytoskeleton 1991; 18(1):41-54.
23. Steinert M, Heuner K. Dictyostelium as host model for pathogenesis. Cell Microbiol 2005; 7(3):307-14.
24. Fajardo M, Schleicher M, Noegel A et al. Calnexin, calreticulin and cytoskeleton-associated proteins modulate uptake and growth of Legionella pneumophila in Dictyostelium discoideum. Microbiology 2004; 150(Pt 9):2825-35.
25. Solomon JM, Leung GS, Isberg RR. Intracellular replication of Mycobacterium marinum within Dictyostelium discoideum: efficient replication in the absence of host coronin. Infect Immun 2003; 71(6):3578-86.
26. Ferrari G, Langen H, Naito M et al. A coat protein on phagosomes involved in the intracellular survival of mycobacteria. Cell 1999; 97(4):435-47.
27. Rybakin V, Clemen CS. Coronin proteins as multifunctional regulators of the cytoskeleton and membrane trafficking. Bioessays 2005; 27(6):625-32.
28. Rybakin V, Stumpf M, Schulze A et al. Coronin 7, the mammalian POD-1 homologue, localizes to the Golgi apparatus. FEBS Lett 2004; 573(1-3):161-7.
29. Mohri K, Vorobiev S, Fedorov AA et al. Identification of functional residues on Caenorhabditis elegans actin-interacting protein 1 (UNC-78) for disassembly of actin depolymerizing factor/cofilin-bound actin filaments. J Biol Chem 2004; 279(30):31697-707.
30. Rybakin V, Gounko NV, Spate K et al. Crn7 interacts with AP-1 and is required for the maintenance of Golgi morphology and protein export from the Golgi. J Biol Chem 2006; 281(41):31070-8.
31. Gloss A, Rivero F, Khaire N et al. Villidin, a novel WD-repeat and villin-related protein from Dictyostelium, is associated with membranes and the cytoskeleton. Mol Biol Cell 2003; 14(7):2716-27.
32. Vardar D, Chishti AH, Frank BS et al. Villin-type headpiece domains show a wide range of F-actin-binding affinities. Cell Motil Cytoskeleton 2002; 52(1):9-21.
33. Fisher PR, Noegel AA, Fechheimer M et al. Photosensory and thermosensory responses in Dictyostelium slugs are specifically impaired by absence of the F-actin cross-linking gelation factor (ABP-120). Curr Biol 1997; 7(11):889-92.
34. Fisher PR. Genetics of phototaxis in a model eukaryote, Dictyostelium discoideum. Bioessays 1997; 19(5):397-407.

35. Asano S, Mishima M, Nishida E. Coronin forms a stable dimer through its C-terminal coiled coil region: an implicated role in its localization to cell periphery. Genes Cells 2001; 6(3):225-35.
36. Arbeitman MN, Furlong EE, Imam F et al. Gene expression during the life cycle of Drosophila melanogaster. Science 2002; 297(5590):2270-5.
37. Bharathi V, Pallavi SK, Bajpai R et al. Genetic characterization of the Drosophila homologue of coronin. J Cell Sci 2004; 117(Pt 10):1911-22.
38. Schulze KL, Broadie K, Perin MS et al. Genetic and electrophysiological studies of Drosophila syntaxin-1A demonstrate its role in nonneuronal secretion and neurotransmission. Cell 1995; 80(2):311-20.
39. Haerry TE, Khalsa O, O'Connor MB et al. Synergistic signaling by two BMP ligands through the SAX and TKV receptors controls wing growth and patterning in Drosophila. Development 1998; 125(20):3977-87.
40. Goode BL, Wong JJ, Butty AC, et al. Coronin promotes the rapid assembly and cross-linking of actin filaments and may link the actin and microtubule cytoskeletons in yeast. J Cell Biol 1999; 144(1):83-98.
41. Rothenberg ME, Rogers SL, Vale RD et al. Drosophila pod-1 crosslinks both actin and microtubules and controls the targeting of axons. Neuron 2003; 39(5):779-91.
42. Marsh L, Letourneau PC. Growth of neurites without filopodial or lamellipodial activity in the presence of cytochalasin B. J Cell Biol 1984; 99(6):2041-7.
43. Bentley D, Toroian-Raymond A. Disoriented pathfinding by pioneer neurone growth cones deprived of filopodia by cytochalasin treatment. Nature 1986; 323(6090):712-5.
44. Bowerman B. Maternal control of pattern formation in early Caenorhabditis elegans embryos. Curr Top Dev Biol 1998; 39:73-117.
45. Aroian RV, Field C, Pruliere G et al. Isolation of actin-associated proteins from Caenorhabditis elegans oocytes and their localization in the early embryo. EMBO J 1997; 16(7):1541-9.
46. Rappleye CA, Paredez AR, Smith CW et al. The coronin-like protein POD-1 is required for anterior-posterior axis formation and cellular architecture in the nematode caenorhabditis elegans. Genes Dev 1999; 13(21):2838-51.
47. Drubin DG, Nelson WJ. Origins of cell polarity. Cell 1996; 84(3):335-44.
48. Tagawa A, Rappleye CA, Aroian RV. Pod-2, along with pod-1, defines a new class of genes required for polarity in the early Caenorhabditis elegans embryo. Dev Biol 2001; 233(2):412-24.
49. Luke-Glaser S, Pintard L, Lu C et al. The BTB protein MEL-26 promotes cytokinesis in C. elegans by a CUL-3-independent mechanism. Curr Biol 2005; 15(18):1605-15.
50. Yonemura I, Mabuchi I. Heterogeneity of mRNA coding for Caenorhabditis elegans coronin-like protein. Gene 2001; 271(2):255-9.
51. Cai L, Makhov AM, Bear JE. F-actin binding is essential for coronin 1B function in vivo. J Cell Sci 2007; 120(Pt 10):1779-90.

Chapter 8

Evolutionary and Functional Diversity of Coronin Proteins

Charles-Peter Xavier, Ludwig Eichinger, M. Pilar Fernandez,
Reginald O. Morgan and Christoph S. Clemen*

Abstract

This chapter discusses various aspects of coronin phylogeny, structure and function that are of specific interest. Two subfamilies of ancient coronins of unicellular pathogens such as *Entamoeba*, *Trypanosoma*, *Leishmania* and *Acanthamoeba* as well as of *Plasmodium*, *Babesia*, and *Trichomonas* are presented in the first two sections. Their coronins generally bind to F-actin and apparently are involved in proliferation, locomotion and phagocytosis. However, there are so far no studies addressing a putative role of coronin in the virulence of these pathogens. The following section delineates genetic anomalies like the chimeric coronin-fusion products with pleckstrin homology and gelsolin domains that are found in amoeba. Moreover, most nonvertebrate metazoa appear to encode CRN8, CRN9 and CRN7 representatives (for these coronin symbols see Chapter 2), but in e.g., *Drosophila melanogaster* and *Caenorhabditis elegans* a CRN9 is missing. The forth section deals with the evolutionary expansion of vertebrate coronins. Experimental data on the F-actin binding CRN2 of *Xenopus* (Xcoronin) including a Cdc42/Rac interactive binding (CRIB) motif that is also present in other members of the coronin protein family are discussed. *Xenopus laevis* represents a case for the expansion of the seven vertebrate coronins due to tetraploidization events. Other examples for a change in the number of coronin paralogs are zebrafish and birds, but (coronin) gene duplication events also occurred in unicellular protozoa. The fifth section of this chapter briefly summarizes three different cellular processes in which CRN4/CORO1A is involved, namely actin-binding, superoxide generation and Ca^{2+}-signaling and refers to the largely unexplored mammalian coronins CRN5/CORO2A and CRN6/CORO2B, the latter binding to vinculin. The final section discusses how, by unveiling the aspects of coronin function in organisms reported so far, one can trace a remarkable evolution and diversity in their individual roles anticipating a rather complex and intricate involvement of coronins in a variety of cellular processes.

Introduction

In the present book a sincere attempt has been made to provide a comprehensive overview on the coronin family of proteins. Other chapters of the book focus on phylogeny, structure, localization and, more interestingly, the roles of coronins in F-actin dynamics through interaction with actin and actin-binding proteins, in vesicular trafficking, in cancer, in certain pathogen virulence and on new possibilities for exploring coronin as an effective drug target. This chapter deals with members of the coronin protein family and specific aspects of coronin function that are not covered in the other chapters.

*Corresponding Author: Christoph S. Clemen—Center for Biochemistry, Medical Faculty, University of Cologne, Joseph-Stelzmann-Str. 52, 50931 Cologne, Germany.
Email: christoph.clemen@uni-koeln.de

The Coronin Family of Proteins, edited by Christoph S. Clemen, Ludwig Eichinger and Vasily Rybakin. ©2008 Landes Bioscience and Springer Science+Business Media.

Currently two synonymous names are mainly used for the different members of the coronin protein family. One is based on a simple numbering system for mammalian coronins 1-7, while the other employs a number-letter system to specify coronins 1A (= 1), 1B (= 2), 1C (= 3), 2A (= 4) and 2B (= 5).[1-3] The current official nomenclature for vertebrate coronins from the HGNC (Human Gene Nomenclature Committee) delineates CORO1A, CORO1B, CORO1C, CORO2A, CORO2B, CORO6 and CORO7 symbols. The process to establish a new and unified nomenclature, which could be based on the one described in Chapter 4 by Reginald O. Morgan and M. Pilar Fernandez, is still in its infancy. Most likely this well-done proposal of a new nomenclature delineating twelve coronin subfamilies (CRN1-CRN12) based on their phylogenetic relationship will be modified by the researchers in the coronin field to preserve some historical aspects. Nevertheless, this chapter will already make use of the symbols of this proposed nomenclature, as the coronin proteins mainly discussed in this chapter, CRN10 and CRN12, are members of the five coronin subfamilies (CRN8, 9, 10, 11, 12) that are unnamed to date. Members of the CRN8 (e.g., *Drosophila* and *Caenorhabditis* short coronins) as well as of the CRN11 family (e.g., the single *Saccharomyces* coronin) are referred to in detail in Chapters 7 (Maria C Shina and Angelika A. Noegel) and 6 (Meghal Gandhi and Bruce L. Goode), respectively. So far no experimental data for a CRN9 family member are available.

In this chapter, we first summarize the published data of coronin proteins from unicellular pathogens: CRN12, the phylogenetically oldest coronin and CRN10, the ancient coronin of alveolata and parabasalids. The *Dictyostelium* short coronin, the first published coronin (see Chapter 3 by Eugenio L. de Hostos), also belongs to the CRN12 family, but is discussed in Chapter 7. In the second part we put forward data on genetic anomalies of non vertebrate coronins, discuss the evolutionary expansion of selected coronins in vertebrates and present some of the data of vertebrate coronins that are not covered in the other chapters. Table 1 provides examples for each of the twelve coronin subfamilies and also includes some basic data on molecular properties, localization and function.

CRN12, the Phylogenetically Oldest Coronin

Members of the CRN12 family are present in Heterolobosea, Euglenozoa and Amoeba. Among these there are a number of human pathogens, like *Entamoeba*, *Trypanosoma*, *Leishmania* and *Acanthamoeba*. In macrophages survival of *Mycobacteria* is mediated by CRN4/CORO1A-dependent activation of calcineurin (see Chapter 10 and Jayachandran et al[4]). This raises the question as to whether coronin might contribute to the pathogenicity of human pathogens.

Acanthamoeba is a medically significant pathogen causing the opportunistic disease granulomatous amoebic encephalitis and the amoebic keratitis of the eye. *A. healyi* Ahcoronin has a predicted molecular mass of 50 kDa and shows significant homology to *D. discoideum* CRN12. An N-terminal EGFP fusion protein of Ahcoronin is localized to the cytosol and the cell periphery with enrichment at the leading edge. Additionally, Ahcoronin transiently localizes to phagocytic cups, however, no enrichment was seen at the mature phagosome.[5] This behaviour resembles the distribution of mammalian CRN4/CORO1A during phagosome maturation (see below) and is an interesting feature to trace the conservation of function. The C-terminus of Ahcoronin (aa 294-454) localized to the cell periphery with an enrichment at the leading edge similar to the full length protein. The EGFP-N terminus (aa 1-49) did not show any specific localization. Similarly, the WD-propeller and the conserved region (aa 50-293) showed a dispersed distribution indicating that the conserved region alone is not involved in actin binding. So far no correlation between pathogenicity and coronin expression in *Acanthamoeba* has been demonstrated. However, since coronin is localized in dynamic areas of the cell, the authors propose that this may indicate the involvement of Ahcoronin in dynamic processes that do require actin-dependent locomotion and phagocytosis.[5]

Leishmania is a protozoan that causes Leishmaniasis. A 56 kDa coronin protein was reported in *Leishmania donovani* that is also a member of the CRN12 subfamily. In immunolabelling studies, N-terminally GFP-tagged *Leishmania* coronin localized to filament-like actin structures in the cell

Table 1. Selected representatives of the coronin subfamilies

Coronin	AA/MW/%I*	Expression/Localization	Function
Acanthamoeba CRN12	454aa, 50kDa, 50%	Cytosol, cell periphery, phagocytic cups, leading edge	Actin-binding protein
Leishmania CRN12	500aa, 56kDa, 28%	Cytosol, filament-like actin structures	Actin-binding protein
Trichomonas CRN10	436aa, 48kDa, 34%	Cell periphery, phagocytic cups and pseudopods	Actin binding protein
Babesia CRN10	573aa, 62kDa, 21%	Cytosol	Actin binding protein
Plasmodium CRN10	372aa, 42kDa, 35%	Cytosol	Actin-binding protein
Dictyostelium Villidin	1704aa, 190kDa, CT homologous to CRN7	Cytosol, Golgi, ER membrane	Actin-binding protein Microtubule-actin linkage
CRN12	445aa, 50kDa, 100%	Cytosol, cortex, Phagocytic cup	Phagocytosis and cytokinesis
CRN7	962aa, 105kDa, 46% homo. to mam.	Actin-rich crown-like CRN3, phagocytic cups	Phagocytosis, structure, leading edge,
Saccharomycetes CRN11	651aa, 72kDa, 57%	Cortical sites of endoctyosis	Coordinates actin dynamics bundling of microtubules and actin linkages
Caenorhabditis CRN8	607aa, 67kDa, 25%	Cytosol, cortex	Establishment of polarity in the developing embryo
CRN7	1057aa, 115kDa, 40%	Actin rich structures at the cell cortex	Establishment of polarity in the developing embryo
Drosophila CRN8	528aa, 57kDa, 54% to Xenopus	Imaginal discs	Mediates trafficking of F-actin coated vesicles and establishment of polarity
CRN7	1074aa, 119kDa, 31% with C. elegans	Enriched in developing axons	Axonal guidance, bundling of microtubules and actin linkages
Xenopus CRN2	480aa, 57kDa, 67%	Cell pheriphery	Actin-binding protein
Human CRN1 (CORO1B)	489aa, 54kDa, 38%	Ubiquitously expressed and localizes to the leading edge of the cell	F-actin turnover by Arp2/3 complex and by cofilin in lamellipodial protrusions

continued on next page

Table 1. Continued

Coronin	AA/MW/%I	Expression/Localization	Function
CRN2 (CORO1C)	474aa, 57kDa, 46%	Cortex, cytosol, leading edge	Actin-binding protein
CRN3 (CORO6)	472aa, 52kDa, 40%	Expressed in brain	N.A.
CRN4 (CORO1A)	461aa, 51kDa, 35%	Cell cortex, cytoplasm, phagosomes of thymocytes, T-cells, macrophages, neutrophils	Activation of Ca^{2+}-dependent signalling reactions, Actin-binding protein
CRN5 (CORO2A)	525aa, 59kDa, 31%	Expressed in brain, epidermis	N.A.
CRN6 (CORO2B)	475aa, 54kDa, 44% with CRN4	Focal adhesions, neurite tips, cell body and stress fibers	Actin and vinculin binding protein
CRN7 (CORO7)	925aa, 104KDa, 29% with Dd CRN7	Expressed in Cytosol, Golgi	Vesicular trafficking

*AA—Number of amino acids, MW—Molecular weight, %I—percent identity with *Dictyostelium* short coronin if not otherwise stated. For *Xenopus* please refer to the text and Tab. 2. There are no experimental data on members of the CRN9 family of coronins present in nonvertebrate metazoa (see Chapter 4).

periphery and uniformly throughout the cytoplasm, but was absent in the flagella. Additionally, the authors reported that ectopical co-expression of *Leishmania* actin and GFP-coronin in mammalian cells induced the formation of filamentous and patch-like structures.[6] *Leishmania* actin and coronin specifically interacted with each other but the interaction was not strong enough to resist the treatment with non-ionic detergents. The leucine zipper motif in *Leishmania* coronin contains five heptads, which suggests the existence of coronin multimers in vivo (see also Chapter 5). Currently, no link between coronin expression and *Leishmania* pathogenicity has been established. However, similar to *Acanthamoeba*, studies investigating a potential role of coronin in the virulence of this pathogen will be interesting and may even open new possibilities for exploiting coronin as drug target.

CRN10, the Ancient Coronin of Alveolata and Parabasalids

Plasmodium falciparum, the major causative agent of human malaria, invades its intermediate host hepatocytes and erythrocytes. The driving force underlying parasite motility and host cell invasion has been suggested to be based on the parasite's actin cytoskeleton.[7-9] *P. falciparum* coronin, a member of the CRN10 family has a calculated mass of 52 kDa and an apparent molecular weight of 42 kDa. It displays 35% identity with *D. discoideum* CRN12 and 27-32% identity with bovine and human coronin. A hallmark for most of the coronins is a leucine zipper motif at the C-terminus which is responsible for di- or multimerization. Surprisingly, this motif apparently is absent in *P. falciparum* CRN10. Cellular fractionation showed *P. falciparum* coronin in the cytosolic and Triton X-100 insoluble fraction. The authors suggest that a better understanding of coronin's role in actin dynamics as well as the identification of additional interacting proteins may help to define molecules critically involved in parasite survival.[10] In this respect it is interesting that CRN10 from *Babesiae bovis, bigemina, divergens* and *canis* cosedimented with actin and was expressed at highest levels during the merozoite stage of this parasite in red blood cells.[11]

Trichomonas vaginalis, the causative agent of the most common nonviral sexually transmitted disease in human known as trichomoniasis, infects 250 to 350 million people worldwide. Trichomoniasis results in serious discomfort to women and is associated with adverse pregnancy outcome, preterm delivery, low-birth-weight infants and fertility, cervical cancer and increase in the transmission of HIV.[12]

A monoclonal antibody raised against a cytoskeletal fraction of *T. vaginalis* identified a closely spaced double-band in SDS-PAGE. The corresponding proteins had an apparent molecular weight of approximately 50 kDa, showed high sequence identity to *D. discoideum* CRN12 and were named Cor1 and Cor2. According to the proposed nomenclature they seem to represent the two CRN10 family members CRN10a and CRN10b that originated by relatively recent lineage-specific gene duplication in *T. vaginalis* (see Chapter 4). The *T. vaginalis* proteins display relatively weak percentage of identity (from 23-33%) with coronins from other organisms. However, this is expected considering the large evolutionary distance between the species.[13] Immunolabelling and electron microscopic studies localized coronin to phagocytic cups and pseudopods of *T. vaginalis* amoeboid cells.[14] Although the whole chain of events leading to host cell lysis remains to be fully elucidated, the authors speculate that coronin might play a major downstream role in a signalling pathway that leads to re-organization of the actin cytoskeleton and the adoption of the amoeboid form of the parasite.[15] The generation of a coronin specific knockout in *T. vaginalis*[16] will be crucial for investigation of this hypothesis. In addition the knock-out cells could be used to study the role of coronin in phagocytosis, pseudopod formation, cell motility and cell proliferation. The knock-out cells should also clarify whether coronin contributes to *T. vaginalis* virulence.

Genetic Anomalies in Nonvertebrate Coronin Proteins

Amoebae such as *Dictyostelium discoideum, Dictyostelium purpureum* and *Entamoeba histolytica* express a unique coronin-villin gene fusion product "villidin" with a presumed dual capacity to influence actin dynamics. The villidin homologs in *D. discoideum* (XP_636652) and *D. purpureum* (scaffold_52) exhibit approx. 82% amino acid identity to each other and approx. 33% amino acid identity with *E. histolytica* putative "villidin" (XP_655366). However, HMM (Hidden Markov Model) analysis revealed no authentic coronin domains in the latter and alignment with the *Dictyostelium* villidin was limited to the C-terminal region. Instead, a distinct actin-binding protein (ABPH, 1602 aa, gb:AF118397) was validated as the true villidin homolog from *E. histolytica*. It contains the coronin DUF1899, two WD40 domains and DUF1900 in its N-terminal region (for the DUF-domains and their contribution to the β-propeller scaffold please refer to Chapter 4) and in addition 3 pleckstrin homology (PH) domains and 3 gelsolin domains in its C-terminal region, similar to its *Dictyostelium* homolog (Fig. 1).

Another interesting anomaly was detected by comparing matched species pairs for the invertebrate CRN8 and CRN9 subfamilies. Most (multicellular) invertebrate species have one representative in each subfamily in addition to a CRN7 representative. Additional searching of substantially complete genomes confirmed some overlooked pairs such as CRN9 (XP_969741) from *Tribolium castaneum* (red flour beetle), however, CRN9 orthologs could not be identified in genomic assembly data for *D. melanogaster* nor *C. elegans*. This indicates some selective gene loss or silencing subsequent to the original gene duplication event in early metazoa. Considering the evolutionary distance between CRN8 and CRN9 members, which share approx. 50% amino acid identity, it is plausible that they retain only limited functional redundancy. Thus the selective CRN9 loss in *Drosophila* and *Caenorhabditis* may be accompanied by measurable phenotypic change when compared to other insect and nematode models.

Evolutionary Expansion of Selected Coronins in Vertebrates

A *X. laevis* homolog of *Dictyostelium* coronin—Xcoronin—has been described as a protein of 480 amino acids with a molecular mass of 57 kDa and 67% identity to human CRN4/CORO1A. Two apparent isoforms were reported for this *X. laevis* coronin, Xcoronin A and B, with 93% identity to each other, capable of forming homo- and hetero-oligomers.[17,18] A recent database analysis identified seven coronins in *X. laevis* and *Xenopus tropicalis*, which are orthologs of the human coronins CRN1-7 with identities between 55 to 84% (see Chapter 4). From these analyses it turned out that Xcoronin A and B both belong to the CRN2 family and, moreover, that CRN2a

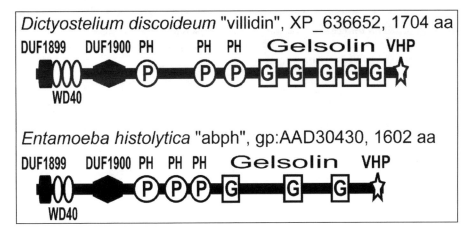

Figure 1. Schematic domain structures are shown for homologous villidin proteins from *D. discoideum* (XP_636652, 1704 aa) and *E. histolytica* ("ABPH", AF118397, 1602 aa). Both contain typical coronin domains at their amino termini in addition to 3 pleckstrin homology (PH), 3-5 gelsolin (G) and a villin headpiece (VHP) domains at the C-termini, all detected by matches to the corresponding hidden Markov models (HMM) from the PFAM database (http://www.sanger.ac.uk/Software/Pfam/).

and CRN2b probably result from a recent whole genome duplication in *X. laevis* (but not *X. tropicalis*) about 40 Mya ago.[19] CRN2a (Xcoronin A) and CRN2b (Xcoronin B) show 94% identity to the single *X. tropicalis* CRN2 copy (BC064872; CORO1C). Thus, *X. tropicalis* (western clawed frog) has seven coronins, i.e., CRN1-CRN7, whereas *X. laevis* (African clawed frog) has at least nine coronins, including duplicates of CRN2/CORO1C and CRN6/CORO2B. Due to the genome duplication *X. laevis* would have been expected to have 14 coronins, i.e., CRN1a-CRN7a and CRN1b and CRN7b, but the missing duplicates may have suffered genetic mishaps during the genome duplication event or may have been silenced (i.e., eroded by mutation) for toxicity or lack of need, as seems to have occurred in teleost fishes like zebrafish (Table 2), that underwent a unique tetraploidization event over 300 million years ago, subsequent to their divergence from jawless and cartilagenous fish. Note that the *X. laevis* CRN2a and CRN2b copies are different from variant isoforms of the same gene, as described for the human CRN2. For human CRN2 (CORO1C) three variants have been detected at the mRNA and protein level (NM_014325, AM849477, AM849478),[20] derived from three transcripts from the same gene by differential splicing. In general, amphibia (e.g., *X. tropicalis*) and reptiles (e.g., the lizard *Anolis carolinensis*) seem to have the full complement of seven vertebrate coronins, whereas birds (e.g., chicken and zebrafinch) possess most coronin loci dispersed in their genomes with the exception of CRN4/CORO1A which has not yet been detected (Table 2). Other organisms that underwent whole genome duplication from a diploid to a tetraploid state include all teleost fishes like medaka and zebrafish, but selective gene duplication and/or extensive gene loss obscure such ancient events in unicellular protozoa like *Cryptosporidium, Trichomonas, Entamoeba* and *Saccharomyces*. The zebrafish genome, for example, has duplicate copies of CRN5/CORO2A, CRN6/CORO2B and CRN2/CORO1C on distinct chromosomes; other coronin duplicates appear to have been lost or silenced (Table 2).

The N- and C- terminal domains of Xcoronin (A and B), CRN2a and CRN2b, were shown to be critical for optimal binding to F-actin.[17] Xcoronin forms a stable dimer via its C-terminal leucine zipper motif. Dimerization of Xcoronin was found to be crucial for its proper colocalization with F-actin at the cell periphery and plays an important role in Rac induced lamellipoidial extensions and cell spreading.[17] However, *X. laevis* CRN2 did not significantly associate with F-actin stress fibres and was absent from focal adhesions and cell-cell contacts unlike CRN5/

Table 2. Coronin repertoires and anomalies in selected vertebrate genomes

Coronin	GenPept	Chromosome	Protein	aa id
Danio rerio (zebrafish) coronin				
CRN4/CORO1A	NP_957408	chr. 3	455 aa	
CRN1/CORO1B	NP_001103177	chr. 7	499 aa	
CRN2a/CORO1C	NP_958452	chr. 5	474 aa	
CRN2b/CORO1C	XP_001341686	chr. 5	474 aa	85%
CRN5a/CORO2A	NP_955937	chr. 1	528 aa	
CRN5b/CORO2A	NP_682841	chr. 23	542 aa	54%
CRN6a/CORO2B	XP_001337394	chr. 25	514 aa	
CRN6b/CORO2B	XP_688721	chr. 7	486 aa	72%
CRN3/CORO6	NP_956690	chr. UN	436 aa	
CRN7/CORO7	NP_001025407	chr. 3	923 aa	
Xenopus laevis (African clawed frog) coronins				
CRN4/CORO1A	NP_001083542		462 aa	
CRN1/CORO1B	jgi:ESTs		partial 233 aa	
CRN2a/CORO1C	NP_001079362		480 aa	
CRN2b/CORO1C	NP_001083772		480 aa	94%
CRN5/CORO2A	NP_001084940		525 aa	
CRN6a/CORO2B	NP_001086406		475 aa	
CRN6b/CORO2B	partial ESTs like BU905412			87%
CRN3/CORO6	(unavailable)		? aa	
CRN7/CORO7	partial ESTs		?aa	
Xenopus tropicalis (western clawed frog) coronins				
CRN4/CORO1A	NP_001005826		459 aa	
CRN1/CORO1B	scaffold_7255		partial 316/489 aa	
CRN2/CORO1C	NP_989353		480 aa	
CRN5/CORO2A	Xentr:352343		524 aa	
CRN6/CORO2B	NP_001016965		475 aa	
CRN3/CORO6	Xentr4:420533		470 aa	
CRN7/CORO7	Xentr:311514		999 aa	
Gallus gallus (chicken) coronins				
CRN4/CORO1A	Present in reptiles (e.g., *Anolis carolinensis*) Not detected in birds			
CRN1/CORO1B	XP_001235734	chr. UN	(partial ug:Gga.23259 aa)	
CRN2/CORO1C	NP_001034354	chr. 15	474 aa	
CRN5/CORO2A	XP_424946	chr. Z	522 aa	
CRN6/CORO2B	NC_006097	chr. 10	475 aa	
CRN3/CORO6	XP_415830	chr. 19	frag.344 aa	
CRN7/CORO7	NP_001006176	chr. 14	923 aa	

The genomes of *Danio rerio* (zebrafish), *X. laevis* (African clawed frog), *X. tropicalis* (western clawed frog) and *Gallus gallus* (chicken) were scanned by BLAST searches to identify their full coronin gene/protein content. The pseudotetraploid genomes of *D. rerio* and *X. laevis* exhibit several duplicate copies for specific genes/proteins that have apparently been retained following known ancient whole genome duplication events in these species. Birds such as chicken and zebrafinch lack CRN4/CORO1A in their present genome assemblies, despite abundant sequence data.

CORO2A.[21] The inability of the dimerization mutants to localize to the cell periphery emphasizes the significance of dimerization for optimal binding to actin filaments as was shown for CRN2/CORO1C.[22] Interestingly, a short sequence stretch that resembles the Cdc42/Rac interactive binding (CRIB) motif was found between amino acids 119 and 134 of *X. laevis* CRN2 and could act as a potential binding site for the activated GTP-binding proteins Rac and Cdc42 involved in the regulation of the actin cytoskeleton.[17,18] Cdc42/Rac effectors contain the conserved CRIB motif that binds the effector domain of Cdc42/Rac GTPases in a GTP-dependent manner.[23,24] Based on the reported CRIB motif in *Xenopus* CRN2 we searched for similar motifs in human coronins and found that this sequence stretch is highly conserved in human CRN4/CORO1A, CRN1/CORO1B, CRN2/CORO1C and CRN3/CORO6, less conserved in human CRN5/CORO2A, CRN6/CORO2B and *Dictyostelium* CRN12 and not conserved in human CRN7/CORO7 (Fig. 2A). In support of a functional role, the CRIB motif is located in a loop which is surface accessible and stretches from β-sheet D of blade 2 with most of the amino acids in the loop region, ending with β-sheet A of blade 3 (Fig. 2B). In Swiss 3T3 cells it has been shown that active Rac induced lamellipodial extension and redistribution of CRN2/CORO1C.[22] Further

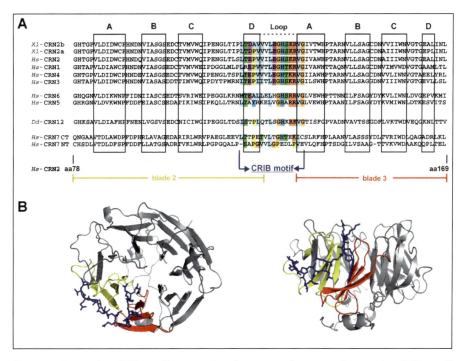

Figure 2. A) Putative CRIB motif in coronins. Sequence alignment of a putative CRIB motif of different *Homo sapiens* coronins (*Hs*-CRN1-7) and *D. discoideum* coronin (*Dd*-CRN12) with *X. laevis* coronins (*Xl*-CRN2a, 2b). Sequence of β-propeller blade 2 (yellow line) and β-propeller blade 3 (red line) corresponding to aa78-169 of *H. sapiens* CORO1C/CRN2 are shown. CRIB motif conservation across different *Human, Dictyostelium* and *Xenopus* coronins is highlighted. Rectangle boxes A-D specify β-strands of the coronin WD domain, the dotted line denotes the loop between blade 2 and 3. B) Structural homology model of coronin 3 (see chapter II-3) highlighting the putative CRIB motif (blue) stretching from β strand D of blade 2 (yellow) and ending with β strand A of blade 3 (red).

experiments should unravel the roles of different coronins in Rac- and Cdc42-mediated signalling to the actin cytoskeleton (Xavier CP, unpublished).

Tissue Specific Expression and Putative Functions of Mammalian Coronins Not Covered in the Other Chapters

The seven mammalian coronins exhibit a distinct pattern of expression across cell types and tissues.[1] The best-characterized CRN4/CORO1A is virtually exclusively expressed in thymocytes, T-cells, macrophages and neutrophils.[25-30] It has been shown to function in actin-dependent processes as well as in specific functions unrelated to actin. For a detailed view on mammalian CORO1A regarding its interaction with actin please refer to Chapters 5 and 6 and to Chapter 11, 5th section, for details regarding actin-unrelated functions please refer to Chapter 10 and also Chapter 11, 5th section.

In order to provide an outline of some of the interesting aspects of mammalian CRN4/CORO1A, three apparently unrelated roles are considered. Firstly, CORO1A has been shown to interact with and regulate F-actin and has been detected in dynamic regions of the submembranous actin cytoskeleton of leucocytes with important implications in the immune system.[27,28,31] A soluble pool of CORO1A in human phagocytic leukocytes forms high-molecular-weight complexes that are solubilized by PI3-kinase activity and may be involved in forming the F-actin structures in early phagosome formation.[32] In addition, ActA-positive *Listeria monocytogenes* have been found to recruit CORO1A to their F-actin tails in infected host cells.[33] Secondly, a putative function reported for CORO1A in the immune system points to the regulation of superoxide generation in connection with a phagocytic vacuole.[30] CORO1A binds C-terminally to p40phox, a cytosolic subunit of the NADPH oxidase complex involved in the generation of the microbicidal superoxide burst in neutrophils. Finally, upon internalization of pathogens like *Mycobacteria*, *Salmonella* and *Heliobacter* as well as of latex beads by macrophages, CORO1A is transiently recruited to the site of entry.[34-38] Whether or not pathogen-derived molecules like lipoamide dehydrogenase C (LpdC) or a cholesterol-specific receptor molecule are involved in this process is currently discussed.[39-41] In contradiction to earlier studies, CORO1A was found dispensable for the phagocytic process itself.[4] Interestingly, the retention of CORO1A on the phagosome inhibits its later fusion with lysosomes and prevents the phagocytosed pathogens from degradation. Here, mechanisms regulating CORO1A transcription,[42] dissociation of CORO1A from the phagosome accompanied by phosphorylation on serine residues involving PKC[43] and calcineurin-signaling[4] may be involved.

A recent study delineated CRN4/CORO1A as an important factor for the development of the autoimmune disease systemic lupus erythematosus (SLE). A spontaneous nonsense mutation of coronin-1A (c.784C>T; p.Gln262X) leading to a truncated and non-functional protein suppressed the development of the autoimmune disease in lupus-prone mice.[44] The mutation led to phenotypes involving the actin cytoskeleton as well as calcium signaling. In this respect the quite different phenotypes observed for the CORO1A knockout mouse strains independently generated by Föger et al[27] and Jayachandran et al[4] are combined in this additional mouse model. Mutated CORO1A resulted in a reduced number of single positive $CD4^+$ and $CD8^+$ T cells, including the naïve and activated subsets, increased rate of apoptosis, decreased proliferation rates, increased levels of cellular F-actin, impaired migration in response to chemokines, and reduced initial calcium entry upon activation.[44] As a consequence of a reduced T helper activity levels of polyclonal serum IgG and anti-dsDNA antibodies were also decreased. Thus, the coronin-1A mutation effectively suppressed cellular as well as humoral manifestations of SLE.[44] These recent data once more emphasize an important role of coronin proteins in, but certainly not limited to, the immune system (see also Chapter 10) as well as development, regeneration and cancer progression (see Chapter 11).

CRN1/CORO1B is ubiquitously expressed at high levels in most of the tissues in contrast to CRN2/CORO1C, which is ubiquitously expressed but at low levels. Three splice variants of CRN3/CORO6 are expressed in the brain (NP_624354, NP_624355, NP_624356). CORO7/CRN7 is ubiquitously expressed but at lower levels compared to other mammalian coronins.

Specific functions of CORO1B, CORO1C and CORO7 are described in their respective chapters (5, 6, 9, 11).

Mammalian CRN5/CORO2A (IR10, ClipinB), a 525 amino acid containing protein, was isolated by screening a human epidermal cDNA library. Northern blot analysis demonstrated high expression levels in brain in addition to lower expression in epidermis, colon, prostate, testis and lung. Studies regarding intracellular localization, F-actin binding and its possible role in F-actin dynamics are yet to be established.[45]

Mammalian CRN6/CORO2B (Clipin C) is one of the predominantly expressed coronin proteins in the nervous system. It is enriched in the brain and expressed at lower levels in other tissues. It consists of 475 aa with a predicted molecular mass of 54 kDa and shows 44% amino acid identity with CORO1A and 61% with CORO2A. Immunocytochemical analysis revealed colocalization of CORO2B with F-actin at focal adhesions, neurite tips and stress fibers. In addition a considerable amount was reported to be dispersed in the cell body. Immunoprecipitation studies showed an association of CORO2B with vinculin, a major component of focal contacts supporting its localization at focal adhesions. In mouse brain CORO2B localized in cerebral cortex, hippocampus, thalamus, olfactory bulb and cerebellum. In the cerebellum the Purkinje cell layer was intensely labeled. Through cosedimentation assays a clear association of CORO2B with F-actin was demonstrated. Altogether the authors propose CORO2B as a possible candidate that would act as a cytoskeleton-membrane connector, implicated in the control of cell adhesions and cell movements in neuronal cells.[21]

Outlook: The Remarkable Functional Diversity of Coronin Proteins

The actin cytoskeleton is one of the most fascinating cellular networks that mediates a variety of essential biological processes critical for the survival of the cell.[46] Its dynamic properties provide the basic force for various processes like cell migration, endocytosis, vesicular trafficking and cytokinesis.[47-49] In order to efficiently execute all these dynamic processes the differential regulation and recruitment of a plethora of actin-binding proteins with distinctive activities is required. One of the major actin binding proteins that has been extensively studied in recent years is coronin.

Coronin was first identified in the social amoeba *D. discoideum* (see Chapter 3). Identification of coronin in other unicellular organisms and higher organisms followed.[1-3] A number of aspects contribute to a rather complex situation for the function of coronin proteins. Firstly, except for F-actin no other binding partner of the WD-domain of coronins has been confirmed yet, even though for other WD-proteins as well as the structurally related Kelch-proteins various interaction partners have been identified (see Chapters 1 and 2). As the WD-propeller domain is regarded as a platform for protein-protein interactions, various binding partners can be anticipated and may disclose a new variety of distinct functions of coronins. Secondly, the C-terminal coiled coil domain of coronins obviously is involved in oligomerization and Arp2/3 binding. Associated with a change in the three-dimensional shape of the coronin molecule are the proper subcellular localization, but also its activity or binding specificity are likely regulated (see Chapter 6). Thirdly, phosphorylation of specific residues in several coronin proteins have been shown to regulate localisation, oligomerization and interaction with other proteins. Possibly, other posttranslational modifications still await detection.

Starting with a single coronin gene in a simple, yet complex eukaryote, the family of coronin proteins expanded to seven paralogues in vertebrates. Gene duplications in some vertebrates might have resulted in up to fourteen different coronin proteins that all might have acquired different cellular functions. In addition, splice variants of mammalian coronins have been detected, that further amplify the functional diversity. By unravelling the cellular functions of coronins in a wide range of organisms, from amoeba to the highly evolved mammals, one can trace a remarkable evolutionary and functional diversity. It is clear that we are only beginning to understand the functional roles of the diverse coronins and we anticipate the involvement of coronins in other cellular processes yet to be explored.

Acknowledgements

We thank Andreas Hofmann for kindly preparing the structural homology models included in Figure 2B (see also Chapter 5). CSC is supported by the DFG (NO 113/13-3) and Köln Fortune. Futhermore, grant supposrts by the Imhoff-and Maria-Pesch-Foundations awarded to CSC are gratefully acknowledged.

References

1. Rybakin V, Clemen CS. Coronin proteins as multifunctional regulators of the cytoskeleton and membrane trafficking. Bioessays 2005; 27(6):625-632.
2. Uetrecht AC, Bear JE. Coronins: the return of the crown. Trends Cell Biol 2006; 16(8):421-426.
3. de Hostos EL. The coronin family of actin-associated proteins. Trends Cell Biol 1999; 9(9):345-350.
4. Jayachandran R, Sundaramurthy V, Combaluzier B et al. Survival of mycobacteria in macrophages is mediated by coronin 1-dependent activation of calcineurin. Cell 2007; 130(1):37-50.
5. Baldo ET, Moon EK, Kong HH et al. Acanthamoeba healyi: molecular cloning and characterization of a coronin homologue, an actin-related protein. Exp Parasitol 2005; 110(2):114-122.
6. Nayak RC, Sahasrabuddhe AA, Bajpai VK et al. A novel homologue of coronin colocalizes with actin in filament-like structures in Leishmania. Mol Biochem Parasitol 2005; 143(2):152-164.
7. Jensen JB, Edgar SA. Possible secretory function of the rhoptries of Eimeria magna during penetration of cultured cells. J Parasitol 1976; 62(6):988-992.
8. Miller LH, Aikawa M, Johnson JG et al. Interaction between cytochalasin B-treated malarial parasites and erythrocytes. Attachment and junction formation. J Exp Med 1979; 149(1):172-184.
9. Ryning FW, Remington JS. Effect of cytochalasin D on Toxoplasma gondii cell entry. Infect Immun 1978; 20(3):739-743.
10. Tardieux I, Liu X, Poupel O et al. A Plasmodium falciparum novel gene encoding a coronin-like protein which associates with actin filaments. FEBS Lett 1998; 441(2):251-256.
11. Figueroa JV, Precigout E, Carcy B et al. Identification of a coronin-like protein in Babesia species. Ann N Y Acad Sci 2004; 1026:125-138.
12. da Costa RF, de Souza W, Benchimol M et al. Trichomonas vaginalis perturbs the junctional complex in epithelial cells. Cell Res 2005; 15(9):704-716.
13. Embley TM, Hirt RP. Early branching eukaryotes? Current opinion in genetics & development 1998; 8(6):624-629.
14. Rendon-Maldonado JG, Espinosa-Cantellano M, Gonzalez-Robles A et al. Trichomonas vaginalis: in vitro phagocytosis of lactobacilli, vaginal epithelial cells, leukocytes and erythrocytes. Exp Parasitol 1998; 89(2):241-250.
15. Bricheux G, Coffe G, Bayle D et al. Characterization, cloning and immunolocalization of a coronin homologue in Trichomonas vaginalis. Eur J Cell Biol 2000; 79(6):413-422.
16. Lehker MW, Benchimol M, Alderete JF. Assigning function to putative virulence genes of Trichomonas vaginalis: utility of targeted, selectable gene-replacement. In: Pandalai SG, ed. Recent Res Devel Microbiology 2004; 8:97-119.
17. Asano S, Mishima M, Nishida E. Coronin forms a stable dimer through its C-terminal coiled coil region: an implicated role in its localization to cell periphery. Genes Cells 2001; 6(3):225-235.
18. Mishima M, Nishida E. Coronin localizes to leading edges and is involved in cell spreading and lamellipodium extension in vertebrate cells. J Cell Sci 1999; 112(Pt 17):2833-2842.
19. Hellsten U, Khokha MK, Grammer TC et al. Accelerated gene evolution and subfunctionalization in the pseudotetraploid frog Xenopus laevis. BMC biology 2007; 5:31.
20. Xavier CP, Rosentreter A, Hofmann A et al. Characterization and functional relevance of coronin 3 isoforms. Submitted for publication.
21. Nakamura T, Takeuchi K, Muraoka S et al. A neurally enriched coronin-like protein, ClipinC, is a novel candidate for an actin cytoskeleton-cortical membrane-linking protein. J Biol Chem 1999; 274(19):13322-13327.
22. Spoerl Z, Stumpf M, Noegel AA et al. Oligomerization, F-actin interaction and membrane association of the ubiquitous mammalian coronin 3 are mediated by its carboxyl terminus. J Biol Chem 2002; 277(50):48858-48867.
23. Aspenstrom P. Effectors for the Rho GTPases. Current opinion in cell biology 1999; 11(1):95-102.
24. Burbelo PD, Drechsel D, Hall A. A conserved binding motif defines numerous candidate target proteins for both Cdc42 and Rac GTPases. The Journal of biological chemistry 1995; 270(49):29071-29074.
25. Suzuki K, Nishihata J, Arai Y et al. Molecular cloning of a novel actin-binding protein, p57, with a WD repeat and a leucine zipper motif. FEBS Lett 1995; 364(3):283-288.
26. Ferrari G, Langen H, Naito M et al. A coat protein on phagosomes involved in the intracellular survival of mycobacteria. Cell 1999; 97(4):435-447.

27. Foger N, Rangell L, Danilenko DM et al. Requirement for coronin 1 in T-lymphocyte trafficking and cellular homeostasis. Science 2006; 313(5788):839-842.
28. Nal B, Carroll P, Mohr E et al. Coronin-1 expression in T-lymphocytes: insights into protein function during T-cell development and activation. Int Immunol 2004; 16(2):231-240.
29. Okumura M, Kung C, Wong S et al. Definition of family of coronin-related proteins conserved between humans and mice: close genetic linkage between coronin-2 and CD45-associated protein. DNA Cell Biol 1998; 17(9):779-787.
30. Grogan A, Reeves E, Keep N et al. Cytosolic phox proteins interact with and regulate the assembly of coronin in neutrophils. J Cell Sci 1997; 110(Pt 24):3071-3081.
31. Yan M, Di Ciano-Oliveira C, Grinstein S et al. Coronin function is required for chemotaxis and phagocytosis in human neutrophils. J Immunol 2007; 178(9):5769-5778.
32. Didichenko SA, Segal AW, Thelen M. Evidence for a pool of coronin in mammalian cells that is sensitive to PI 3-kinase. FEBS Lett 2000; 485(2-3):147-152.
33. David V, Gouin E, Troys MV et al. Identification of cofilin, coronin, Rac and capZ in actin tails using a Listeria affinity approach. J Cell Sci 1998; 111(Pt 19):2877-2884.
34. Schuller S, Neefjes J, Ottenhoff T et al. Coronin is involved in uptake of Mycobacterium bovis BCG in human macrophages but not in phagosome maintenance. Cell Microbiol 2001; 3(12):785-793.
35. Zheng PY, Jones NL. Helicobacter pylori strains expressing the vacuolating cytotoxin interrupt phagosome maturation in macrophages by recruiting and retaining TACO (coronin 1) protein. Cell Microbiol 2003; 5(1):25-40.
36. Suzuki K, Takeshita F, Nakata N et al. Localization of CORO1A in the Macrophages Containing Mycobacterium leprae. Acta Histochem Cytochem 2006; 39(4):107-112.
37. Yan M, Collins RF, Grinstein S et al. Coronin-1 function is required for phagosome formation. Mol Biol Cell 2005; 16(7):3077-3087.
38. Garin J, Diez R, Kieffer S et al. The phagosome proteome: insight into phagosome functions. J Cell Biol 2001; 152(1):165-180.
39. Deghmane AE, Soulhine H, Bach H et al. Lipoamide dehydrogenase mediates retention of coronin-1 on BCG vacuoles, leading to arrest in phagosome maturation. J Cell Sci 2007; 120(Pt 16):2796-2806.
40. Gatfield J, Pieters J. Essential role for cholesterol in entry of mycobacteria into macrophages. Science 2000; 288(5471):1647-1650.
41. Kaul D, Anand PK, Verma I. Cholesterol-sensor initiates M. tuberculosis entry into human macrophages. Mol Cell Biochem 2004; 258(1-2):219-222.
42. Anand PK, Kaul D, Sharma M. Green tea polyphenol inhibits Mycobacterium tuberculosis survival within human macrophages. Int J Biochem Cell Biol 2006; 38(4):600-609.
43. Itoh S, Suzuki K, Nishihata J et al. The role of protein kinase C in the transient association of p57, a coronin family actin-binding protein, with phagosomes. Biol Pharm Bull 2002; 25(7):837-844.
44. Haraldsson MK, Louis-Dit-Sully CA, Lawson BR, et al. The Lupus-related Lmb3 Locus Contains a disease-suppressing Coronin-1A Gene Mutation. Immunity. 2008:In press.
45. Zaphiropoulos PG, Toftgard R. cDNA cloning of a novel WD repeat protein mapping to the 9q22.3 chromosomal region. DNA Cell Biol. Dec 1996;15(12):1049-1056.
46. Drubin DG, Nelson WJ. Origins of cell polarity. Cell. Feb 9 1996;84(3):335-344.
47. Satterwhite LL, Pollard TD. Cytokinesis. Current opinion in cell biology. Feb 1992;4(1):43-52.
48. Stossel TP. On the crawling of animal cells. Science New York, N.Y. May 21 1993;260(5111):1086-1094.
49. Mitchison TJ, Cramer LP. Actin-based cell motility and cell locomotion. Cell. Feb 9 1996;84(3):371-379.

CHAPTER 9

Role of Mammalian Coronin 7 in the Biosynthetic Pathway

Vasily Rybakin*

Abstract

Most coronin proteins rely on interaction with actin in their functions. Mammalian coronin 7 has not been shown to interact with actin, but rather to bind to the outer side of Golgi complex membranes. Targeting of coronin 7 to Golgi membranes requires the activity of Src kinase and integrity of AP-1 adaptor protein complex. Coronin 7 further physically interacts with both AP-1 and Src in vivo and in vitro and is phosphorylated by Src. Depletion of coronin 7 by RNAi results in Golgi breakdown and accumulation of arrested cargo proteins, suggesting the protein functions in the later stages of cargo sorting and export from the Golgi complex. We suggest that coronin 7 acts as a mediator of cargo vesicle formation at the trans-Golgi network (TGN) downstream of AP-1 interaction with cargo but upstream of protein kinase D dependent membrane fission.

Introduction

The ability to bind actin is an intrinsic capacity of coronin proteins (reviewed in refs. 1, 2). In some family members, it is often hard to define the bona fide actin binding domain because most parts of the molecule possess actin binding properties.[3-5] There is at least one family member, however, which until to date has not been shown to physically interact or colocalize with actin. Although it is quite possible that future research will reveal specific conditions, processes or cell types where mammalian coronin 7 (CRN7; current official symbol: CORO7) associates with actin cytoskeleton, the current data suggest that this family member is unique in that its function is irrelevant to the regulation of the cytoskeleton.

Molecular Architecture

Coronin 7 belongs to the subgroup of "longer", i.e., double-core coronins.[1] The human protein consists of 925 amino acids and displays a molecular architecture similar to that of *Drosophila melanogaster* and *Caenorhabditis elegans* POD-1 proteins (Fig. 1A). It is 46% and 47% homologous and 30% and 29% identical to *Drosophila* Dpod-1 and *C. elegans* POD-1, respectively. The regions of highest homology to the predicted seven-blade propeller structure[6] of murine coronin 1 (coronin 1A, p57) correspond to amino acids 7-344 and 471-815 in human coronin 7, implying a double seven-blade propeller. The unique feature of the human coronin 7 is a 47 amino acid long low complexity proline-, serine- and threonine-enriched region in the intermediate region of the molecule (amino acids 425-472), N-terminal to the second propeller. Like both POD-1 coronins, mammalian coronin 7 lacks the C-terminal coiled-coil domain. There are no predicted transmembrane domains or signal peptide sequences.

*Vasily Rybakin—The Scripps Research Institute, 10550 N Torrey Pines Rd, Mail Stop IMM1, La Jolla, California 92037, USA. Email: vrybakin@scripps.edu

The Coronin Family of Proteins, edited by Christoph S. Clemen, Ludwig Eichinger and Vasily Rybakin. ©2008 Landes Bioscience and Springer Science+Business Media.

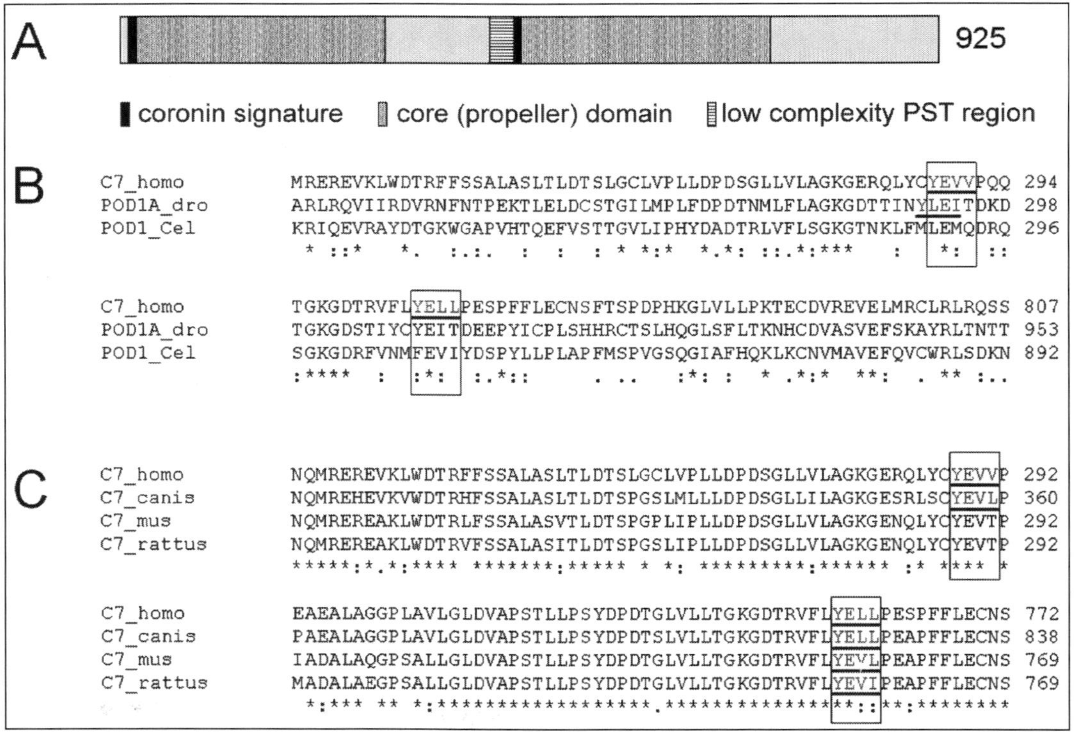

Role of Mammalian Coronin 7 in the Biosynthetic Pathway

A

■ coronin signature ▦ core (propeller) domain ▨ low complexity PST region

925

B

```
C7_homo    MREREVKLWDTRFFSSALASLTLDTSLGCLVPLLDPDSGLLVLAGKGERQLYCYEVVPQQ  294
POD1A_dro  ARLRQVIIRDVRNFNTPEKTLELDCSTGILMPLFDPDTNMLFLAGKGDTTINVLEITDKD  298
POD1_Cel   KRIQEVRAYDTGKWGAPVHTQEFVSTTGVLIPHYDADTRLVFLSGKGTNKLFMLEMQDRQ  296
           * ::*    :   .:..  :       :  *.*:  ::.:*:**  :   ::

C7_homo    TGKGDTRVFLYELLPESPFFLECNSFTSPDPHKGLVLLPKTECDVREVELMRCLRLRQSS  807
POD1A_dro  TGKGDSTIYCYEITDEEPYICPLSHHRCTSLHQGLSFLTKNHCDVASVEFSKAYRLTNTI  953
POD1_Cel   SGKGDRFVNMFEVIYDSPYLLPLAPFMSPVGSQGIAFHQKLKCNVMAVEFQVCWRLSDKN  892
           :*****  :  :*:: :    : .   ::*      *.*:*  **:   . ** :..
```

C

```
C7_homo    NQMREREVKLWDTRFFSSALASLTLDTSLGCLVPLLDPDSGLLVLAGKGERQLYCYEVVP  292
C7_canis   NQMREHEVKVWDTRHFSSALASLTLDTSPGSLMLLLDPDSGLLILAGKGESRLSCYEVLP  360
C7_mus     NQMREREAKLWDTRLFSSALASVTLDTSPGPLIPLLDPDSGLLVLAGKGENQLYCYEVTP  292
C7_rattus  NQMREREAKLWDTRVFSSALASITLDTSPGSLIPLLDPDSGLLVLAGKGENQLYCYEVTP  292
           *****:* *:***:.***:*****.**:*  :  ***:****:** ****.:: **. *

C7_homo    EAEALAGGPLAVIGLDVAPSTLLPSYDPDTGLVLLTGKGDTRVFLYELLPESPFFLECNS  772
C7_canis   PAEALAGGPLAVIGLDVAPSTLLPSYDPDTSLVLLTGKGDTRVFLYELLPEAPFFLECNS  838
C7_mus     IADALAQGPSALLGLDVAPSTLLPSYDPDTGLVLLTGKGDTRVFLYEVLPEAPFFLECNS  769
C7_rattus  MADALAEGPSALLGLDVAPSTLLPSYDPDTGLVLLTGKGDTRVFLYEVIPEAPFFLECNS  769
           :***:* ** :::**************** **************:** ***:.*****
```

Figure 1. Molecular architecture and phylogenetic analysis of coronin 7 proteins. A), Domain structure of human coronin 7. Core domains consisting of WD repeats are preceded by "coronin signature" motifs.[1] Note the low complexity proline, serine- and threonine-enriched domain preceding the second core. B), Partial comparison of amino acid sequences of human coronin 7 (top), *Drosophila* POD1 isoform A (middle) and *C. elegans* POD-1 (bottom). Predicted YxxΦ motifs are highlighted in gray and boxed. C), Partial comparison of amino acid sequences of human, dog, mouse and rat coronin 7 (top to bottom). Predicted YxxΦ motifs are highlighted in gray and boxed. See text for details.

Software predictions[7-9] suggest a number of potential phosphorylation sites in the coronin 7 protein. The highest E value predictions are for potential MAP kinase phosphorylation sites at serine residue 442 and threonines 497 and 733, cdc2 sites at S-450 and S-775, cdk5 at S-437, PKC sites at S-7, S-465 and T-654 and Src sites at tyrosine residues 288 and 758. Not surprisingly, many serine and threonine phosphorylation predictions concentrate in the low complexity PST-enriched region. Although it remains to be elucidated which of the predicted sites are relevant in vivo, at least some of them have been experimentally demonstrated to be phosphorylated in vitro (see below).

Tissue Distribution and Subcellular Localization

Coronin 7 has been detected in most murine tissues by western blot, with the notable exception of heart and skeletal muscle, and the corresponding mRNA was found to be strongly enriched in the brain, kidney and thymus.[10] In cultured mammalian cells, the protein is easily detected by immunofluorescence in the Golgi/TGN area partially colocalizing with both Golgi and TGN markers and this localization is abolished in cells treated with brefeldin A, a fungal metabolite known to fuse Golgi membranes with endoplasmic reticulum.[10,11] Additional analyses revealed that coronin 7 resides at the outer side of Golgi membranes where it could be detected by immunoelectron microscopy (VR, unpublished observations). Additionally, the protein is not protected from proteolytic cleavage by the compartment membrane (Rybakin et al, submitted for publication).

A substantial amount of coronin 7 is additionally present in unidentified cytoplasmic "spots" probably corresponding to large protein complexes or very small vesicles of unknown nature. Subcellular fractionation experiments showed that the bulk of the protein is actually cytosolic and only a minor fraction coincides with a detergent-soluble membrane pellet. Interestingly, in contrast to the cytosolic pool, membrane-associated coronin 7 was found to be phosphorylated on tyrosine residues, as demonstrated by two-dimensional gel electrophoresis and western blot with anti-phosphotyrosine antibodies.[10] This finding led to the conclusion that tyrosine phosphorylation may either be required for membrane targeting of coronin 7 or for its function on membranes. As discussed above, the strongest predicted tyrosine phosphorylation sites were found at tyrosine residues 288 and 758.

In vitro phosphorylation experiments have been performed in order to find out whether predicted phosphorylation sites are biologically relevant. Because tyrosine phosphorylation has been shown to coincide with membrane localization of coronin 7, various tyrosine kinase activities were tested for their ability to influence coronin 7 targeting. Firstly, it has been established that nonspecific inhibition of tyrosine protein kinases resulted in the decrease in membrane-bound coronin 7. Additionally, SU6656, a specific inhibitor of Src family kinases showed the same effect; moreover, it has been demonstrated that expression of dominant negative Src resulted in the redistribution of coronin 7 to the cytosol (Rybakin et al, submitted for publication). These data suggested that Src kinase activity may be required to bring coronin 7 to membranes. Further experiments showed that purified recombinant Src was able to specifically phosphorylate tyrosine 288 as well as 758 of synthetic coronin 7 peptides and phosphorylation of tyrosine 758 was significantly stronger than that of tyrosine 288. Full-length recombinant coronin 7 also is phosphorylated by purified Src in vitro. Additionally, endogenous Src and coronin 7 could be co-immunoprecipitated from HeLa cells (Rybakin et al, submitted for publication). Together, these data suggest that phosphorylation of coronin 7 by Src may be a key mechanism regulating the recruitment of coronin 7 from the cytosol to Golgi membranes.

The Function of Coronin 7 in the Biosynthetic Pathway

The Golgi complex is the central protein sorting organelle in mammalian cells. Total protein input from the endoplasmic reticulum reaches the cis-side of the compartment and cargo proteins gradually traverse the Golgi while being sequentially modified. It is believed that protein modification, most importantly glycosylation, provides cargo proteins with "sorting signals" which are recognized by luminal binding sites of cargo receptors and define the Golgi export route that the cargo will take. Additional sorting clues are provided by short amino acid motifs exposed to the cytosolic side of the Golgi membrane. Upon reaching the trans-Golgi network, cargo proteins are sorted into distinct subpopulations of transport intermediates according to their sorting signals.

The Golgi localization of coronin 7 and its interaction with the sorting machinery suggested that the protein could participate in the regulation of protein trafficking along the biosynthetic pathway. RNAi experiments demonstrated that transient depletion of coronin 7 is sufficient for an effective inhibition of protein export from the Golgi. An anterograde trafficking marker, vesicular stomatitis virus glycoprotein G (VSVG), has been shown to accumulate in the Golgi/TGN zone and its further transport is severely affected. Quantification of VSVG fluorescence at the cell surface showed that indeed most of the protein does not reach plasma membrane upon coronin 7 RNAi. Apart from protein trafficking defects, cells treated with coronin 7 siRNA exhibit marked defects in Golgi morphology.[11] As shown by immunofluorescence and electron microscopy, perinuclear Golgi ribbons are disintegrated and short mini-stacks positive for both cis- and trans-Golgi markers are scattered throughout the cytosol. A similar morphology has been previously described in cells treated with the microtubule depolymerizing agent nocodazole. However, in nocodazole treated cells cargo progression is not perturbed.[12] It is highly unlikely that trafficking defects in coronin 7 RNAi cells are due to ineffective or incomplete glycosylation. In RNAi experiments, the marker cargo protein LAMP1[13,14] has been shown to be properly glycosylated in the absence of coronin 7, while a knockdown of a COG3 protein known to participate in the glycosylation in the Golgi[15] resulted in the decrease of LAMP1 glycosylation.[11]

Because of the lack of a signal peptide or hydrophobic regions, coronin 7 protein is likely to be linked to the outer side of the compartment membrane by means of interaction with another membrane protein or proteins. This assumption has been experimentally confirmed by the finding that coronin 7 interacts with the AP-1 adaptor protein complex in vivo and in vitro.[11] The heterotetrameric AP-1 complex associates with cytosolic tails of biosynthetic cargo and cargo receptors en route from the TGN to late endosomes and lysosomes. μ-subunits of AP complexes are known to specifically bind to YxxΦ motifs present in cytosolic tails of AP-1 cargo molecules.[16] Interestingly, coronin 7 possesses two YxxΦ motifs located in the C-terminal parts of each WD repeat propeller (288-291, 758-761) and is therefore theoretically capable of interacting with AP-1 via its μ1 subunit. Indeed, coronin 7 was detected in complex with AP-1 precipitated using an antibody recognizing γ1-adaptin and, reversely, γ1-adaptin was detected coprecipitated together with coronin 7. Additionally, direct and specific interaction between peptides harboring coronin 7 YxxΦ motifs and purified μ1 has been demonstrated in surface plasmon resonance experiments. The predicted sorting motif based on tyrosine 288 showed the strongest binding to the AP-1μ subunit.[11]

The interaction with the AP-1 complex appears biologically significant because in coronin 7 RNAi cells, the AP-1 dependent cargo molecule mannose-6-phosphate receptor MPR46 is accumulated in the Golgi zone and this accumulation coincides with increased AP-1 staining at the TGN.[11] Depletion of μ1-adaptin resulted in the dispersal of coronin 7 from Golgi membranes (Rybakin et al, submitted for publication) implying that the integrity of AP-1 and its membrane localization is indeed required for the Golgi targeting of coronin 7. It is reasonable to believe that coronin 7 functions immediately downstream of the cargo binding to the AP-1 complex, allowing the transport intermediate to form and/or detach.

Coronin 7 Mediated Regulation of Golgi Function: Species-Specific Mechanisms?

It has been convincingly demonstrated that the mammalian coronin 7 is localized to the Golgi complex and regulates protein traffic in the anterograde direction.[10,11] Chapter 7 summarizes the functions of invertebrate coronin 7 orthologs. Indeed, there is evidence that nonmammalian orthologs may function in the biosynthetic pathway as well. This is best illustrated by the *C. elegans* phenotype where POD-1 (coronin 7) deletion results in defects in the formation of the embryonic eggshell and accumulation of vesicular structures within the egg. It has been shown that in mammalian cells, two critical residues are essential for the interaction of coronin 7 with the AP-1 complex and Src protein kinase. Tyrosine 288-basedsignal appears to be the key motif for binding of coronin 7 to the μ subunit of AP-1,[11] while tyrosine 758 is the crucial Src phosphorylation site (Rybakin et al, submitted for publication). Are these residues conserved?

Phylogenetic analysis (Fig. 1B) demonstrates that the conservation of the amino acid sequences in the vicinity of tyrosines 288 and 758 among invertebrates is very low. Although the *Drosophila* sequence features a slightly shifted YxxΦ motif not identical to that of human coronin 7, there is no YxxΦ motif at the vicinity of the residue 288 in the *C. elegans* POD-1 sequence. Moreover, the Src target tyrosine Y758 in the human sequence is conserved in *Drosophila* but absent in *C. elegans*. This suggests that the coronin 7 ortholog in *Drosophila* may be similar to the human protein as far as its regulation is concerned, but the worm ortholog appears to function in a different manner and/or to be completely differently regulated.

Interestingly, although coronin 7 proteins are very well conserved among mammalian species, both tyrosine residues implicated in the regulation of coronin 7 are located in higher variability regions (Fig. 1C). Although the tyrosine 758 is well conserved as well as its vicinity, the tyrosine-based YxxΦ motif at tyrosine 288 is not present in the mouse and rat protein sequence because of the change in the fourth (Φ) amino acid. Interestingly, the YxxΦ motif based on tyrosine 758 shown to bind to μ1 albeit with a lower affinity than tyrosine 288[11] is well conserved in most mammalian species including mouse and rat and may indeed participate in the binding to the adaptor complex. It will be interesting to decipher the relationship between the phosphorylation by Src and binding to AP-1 in the case of tyrosine 758. It may well be possible that phosphorylation will dramatically increase the affinity of AP-1 to the conserved tyrosine 758-based sorting signal.

Future Directions

The exact mechanism that is involved in the coronin 7 mediated regulation of cargo exit from the Golgi complex remains to be elucidated. One of several possible mechanisms includes a role in the formation of a clathrin cage around the AP-1 complexed with cargo. Future experiments will need to address the question whether there is a clathrin coat accumulating in Golgi remnants in coincidence with arrested cargo and AP-1. Additionally, it has been suggested that coronin 7 may be a part of the protein kinase D related machinery regulating the formation of basolateral transport intermediates at the TGN.[17,18] It is unclear how the AP-1/clathrin system interacts with PKD-dependent mechanisms of transport carrier formation and it is not even clear whether the two ever participate in the regulation of the formation of the same vesicle. It has, however, been established that at least basolateral protein transport in polarized cells requires both protein kinase D activity[18] and adaptor protein complexes.[19,20] Coronin 7 may constitute the missing link between the AP complex binding to the cargo at the TGN and activation of diacylglycerol-dependent recruitment and subsequent activation of PKD resulting in the membrane fission.

References

1. Rybakin V, Clemen CS. Coronin proteins as multifunctional regulators of the cytoskeleton and membrane trafficking. Bioessays 2005; 27(6):625-632.
2. Uetrecht AC, Bear JE. Coronins: the return of the crown. Trends Cell Biol 2006; 16(8):421-426.
3. Liu CZ, Chen Y, Sui SF. The identification of a new actin-binding region in p57. Cell Res 2006; 16(1):106-112.
4. Oku T, Itoh S, Okano M et al. Two regions responsible for the actin binding of p57, a mammalian coronin family actin-binding protein. Biol Pharm Bull 2003; 26(4):409-416.
5. Spoerl Z, Stumpf M, Noegel AA et al. Oligomerization, F-actin interaction and membrane association of the ubiquitous mammalian coronin 3 are mediated by its carboxyl terminus. J Biol Chem 2002; 277(50):48858-48867.
6. Appleton BA, Wu P, Wiesmann C. The crystal structure of murine coronin-1: a regulator of actin cytoskeletal dynamics in lymphocytes. Structure 2006; 14(1):87-96.
7. Wong YH, Lee TY, Liang HK et al. KinasePhos 2.0: a web server for identifying protein kinase-specific phosphorylation sites based on sequences and coupling patterns. Nucleic Acids Res 2007; 35(Web Server issue):W588-594.

8. Huang HD, Lee TY, Tzeng SW et al. KinasePhos: a web tool for identifying protein kinase-specific phosphorylation sites. Nucleic Acids Res 2005; 33(Web Server issue):W226-229.
9. Blom N, Sicheritz-Ponten T, Gupta R et al. Prediction of posttranslational glycosylation and phosphorylation of proteins from the amino acid sequence. Proteomics 2004; 4(6):1633-1649.
10. Rybakin V, Stumpf M, Schulze A et al. Coronin 7, the mammalian POD-1 homologue, localizes to the Golgi apparatus. FEBS Lett 2004; 573(1-3):161-167.
11. Rybakin V, Gounko NV, Spate K et al. Crn7 interacts with AP-1 and is required for the maintenance of Golgi morphology and protein export from the Golgi. J Biol Chem 2006; 281(41):31070-31078.
12. Trucco A, Polishchuk RS, Martella O et al. Secretory traffic triggers the formation of tubular continuities across Golgi sub-compartments. Nat Cell Biol 2004; 6(11):1071-1081.
13. D'Souza MP, August JT. A kinetic analysis of biosynthesis and localization of a lysosome-associated membrane glycoprotein. Arch Biochem Biophys 1986; 249(2):522-532.
14. Guarnieri FG, Arterburn LM, Penno MB et al. The motif Tyr-X-X-hydrophobic residue mediates lysosomal membrane targeting of lysosome-associated membrane protein 1. J Biol Chem 1993; 268(3):1941-1946.
15. Shestakova A, Zolov S, Lupashin V. COG complex-mediated recycling of Golgi glycosyltransferases is essential for normal protein glycosylation. Traffic 2006; 7(2):191-204.
16. Robinson MS. Adaptable adaptors for coated vesicles. Trends Cell Biol 2004; 14(4):167-174.
17. Liljedahl M, Maeda Y, Colanzi A et al. Protein kinase D regulates the fission of cell surface destined transport carriers from the trans-Golgi network. Cell 2001; 104(3):409-420.
18. Yeaman C, Ayala MI, Wright JR et al. Protein kinase D regulates basolateral membrane protein exit from trans-Golgi network. Nat Cell Biol 2004; 6(2):106-112.
19. Simmen T, Honing S, Icking A et al. AP-4 binds basolateral signals and participates in basolateral sorting in epithelial MDCK cells. Nat Cell Biol 2002; 4(2):154-159.
20. Ang AL, Taguchi T, Francis S et al. Recycling endosomes can serve as intermediates during transport from the Golgi to the plasma membrane of MDCK cells. J Cell Biol 2004; 167(3):531-543.

CHAPTER 10

Coronin 1 in Innate Immunity

Jean Pieters*

Abstract

The WD repeat containing family of coronin proteins is generally referred to as F-actin-interacting proteins. While in lower eukaryotes such as *Dictyostelium discoideum*, the single short coronin protein regulates several F-actin dependent processes such as motility, phagocytosis and macropinocytosis, the function of any of the seven coronin isoforms in mammals is far less understood. This chapter describes the current knowledge on mammalian coronin 1 (coronin 1A), the closest homologue to *Dictyostelium* short coronin that is exclusively expressed in leukocytes. Recent work based on biochemical, molecular biological and genetic analysis suggest that coronin 1 has evolved a function that is quite different from the F-actin regulatory function of *Dictyostelium* short coronin. Rather, mammalian coronin 1 is involved in the regulation of leukocyte specific signaling events.

Introduction

Almost twenty years ago, a protein was isolated from the social amoeba *Dictyostelium discoideum* that was purified from precipitated actin/myosin complexes. Antibodies against this protein decorated the crown-shaped surface projections of growth phase *Dictyostelium* cells and hence the protein was termed 'coronin'.[1] The finding that coronin cosediments with F-actin in vitro and that a *Dictyostelium* mutant lacking coronin shows reduced motility and phagocytosis, both of which are dependent on F-actin, prompted the designation of coronin as an actin binding protein. The most striking feature of *Dictyostelium* coronin is the presence of a large, central WD (Tryp-Asp) repeat domain linked to a C-terminal coiled coil region. As a consequence, when mammalian proteins were identified harboring a similar central WD repeat followed by a coiled coil domain, they were referred to as members of the actin-binding protein family of coronins.

This chapter presents a different view for coronin 1 (coronin 1A), which is a leukocyte-specific, WD repeat containing protein with ~35% homology to *Dictyostelium* short coronin.[2,3] Based on experimental evidence that will be discussed below, it will be argued that coronin 1 has a function unrelated to the regulation of F-actin dynamics, instead functioning in the regulation of leukocyte signaling processes.

Coronins from Unicellular Organisms

The identification of coronin in *Dictyostelium* was followed by the characterization of a coronin-related molecule in yeast.[4] Unlike *Dictyostelium* that harbors three coronins, the single short coronin as well as a coronin 7 homologue (corA) and villidin (see Chapter 7), yeast contains a single coronin gene, termed *crn1*. Although, yeast coronin interacts with Arp2/3 in vitro,[5] in contrast to the deletion of the short coronin in *Dictyostelium*, *crn1*-null mutants do not have any obvious phenotype and display normal F-actin dynamics.[4]

*Jean Pieters—Biozentrum, University of Basel, Klingelbergstrasse 70, CH 4056 Basel, Switzerland. Email: jean.pieters@unibas.ch

The Coronin Family of Proteins, edited by Christoph S. Clemen, Ludwig Eichinger and Vasily Rybakin. ©2008 Landes Bioscience and Springer Science+Business Media.

Coronins in Multicellular Invertebrate Organisms

Not much is known on the biology of coronins in the multicellular organisms *Caenorhabditis elegans* and *Drosophila melanogaster*. In *C. elegans*, a molecule named POD-1 that contains two stretches of WD repeats but no coiled coils, may be involved in the establishment of polarity in the developing embryo.[6] In Drosophila, a Pod-1 homologue plays a role in axonal growth cone targeting.[7] Besides Pod-1, both *C. elegans* as well as *D. melanogaster* contain a gene that encodes a protein (coro) that is far closer to *Dictyostelium* short coronin than Pod-1. However, while several *Drosophila* deletion mutants lacking coro show a rather pleiotropic phenotype, no information is available on a function for *C. elegans* coronin.

Mammalian Coronin 1

Coronin 1 (coronin 1A) is exclusively expressed in mammalian leukocytes, with no detectable expression in any other cell type ([3] and data not shown). Several other coronin isoforms are expressed as well in leukocytes and therefore coronin 1 may have evolved to perform a highly specialized function in leukocytes. Interestingly, of all mammalian coronin isoforms, coronin 1 is the closest homologue to *Dictyostelium* short coronin. Whether or not the other coronin isoforms have evolved from coronin 1 or have arisen through a different evolutionary path is discussed to in Chapter 4.

Structure of Coronin 1

Coronin 1 Has a Three-Domain Structure

A detailed sequence analysis revealed that coronin 1 (coronin 1A) is made up of three distinct domains (see Fig. 1A): The first, N terminal domain that also contains the 5 WD repeats is rich in β-sheet and is referred to as β–propeller (residues 1-355). The second domain is comprised of a region with little regular secondary structure and is referred to as linker domain (residues 356-429). Finally, the third domain is a coiled coil containing segment which is rich in α-helices (residues 430-461).[8]

The Coronin 1 N-Terminal Domain Contains a 7-Bladed Propeller

One of the characteristic structure of all coronins are their central WD40 domains (see ref. 9 and Chapters 2 and 5). These repeats are characterized by a ~30-40 amino acid residue segment that are bordered by Gly-His (GH) and Trp-Asp (WD) peptide residues.[10,11] The WD repeat unit was first recognized in the beta subunit of the GTP binding protein transducin.[12] This domain seems to have evolved with the eukaryotic kingdom and may be involved in protein:protein interactions, although the precise function of the WD repeat domains in many proteins remains unknown.[13,14]

Coronin-1 possesses 5 WD repeats and based on the homology with the G protein beta subunits it has been proposed that the WD repeat folds into a 5-bladed beta propeller.[9] However, an extensive sequence analysis of coronin 1 revealed the presence of two additional sequence stretches of 46 and 44 residues, respectively, that flank the WD repeat-containing core sequence and are predicted to form four short β-strands and align with the corresponding β-strands of the five WD repeats.[8] Since WD repeats are not strictly necessary to assert a propeller fold,[15-17] the prediction suggests that the coronin 1 propeller domain is, in fact, made up of at least seven blades instead of the previously proposed five blades.[8] Consistent with this analysis, the crystal structure of coronin 1 indeed revealed the presence of a 7-bladed propeller[18] (see Fig. 1B,C). Furthermore, the presence of a 7-bladed propeller in coronin 1 is consistent with the predicted similarity between the coronin 1 N-terminal domain and the yeast transcriptional repressor Tup1[19] as well as the G protein β-subunit,[20] both WD repeat containing seven-bladed β-propeller proteins.

Coronin 1 Assembles into Coiled Coil Mediated Trimers

The C-terminal coiled coil in coronin 1 had been generally assumed to be involved in dimerization.[9] However, observation of purified coronin 7 molecules isolated from macrophages by transmission electron microscopy revealed uniformly distributed particles with an apparent

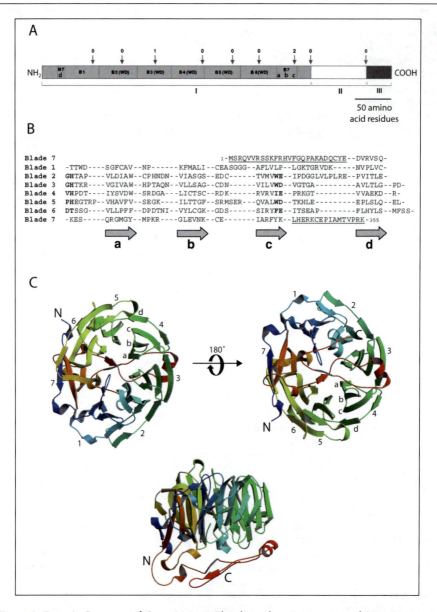

Figure 1. Domain Structure of Coronin 1. A) The three domain structure of coronin 1 (coronin 1A). The N-terminal, 7-bladed beta propeller region consist of 5 typical WD repeats complemented with two stretches of sequence each forming four short β strands, representing two additional blades of the propeller. The propeller region is followed by a linker region. The C-terminal part of coronin 1 is composed of a coiled coil. B) Secondary structure prediction suggests a seven-bladed β-propeller fold reminiscent of the ones of the yeast transcriptional repressor Tup1 and β-subunit of the G protein. The GlyHis and TrpAsp dipeptides of the five WD repeats are highlighted in bold. Predicted blade numbers and corresponding β-strands (gray arrows) are shown on the left and on the bottom of the alignment, respectively. The N- and C-terminal domain extensions are underlined. C) Model of coronin 1 lacking the coiled coil domain based on the X-ray structure. From[8] (A,B) and[18] (C).

three-fold symmetry (Fig. 2). Further biochemical analysis suggested that the observed lobes apparent in Figure 2 correspond to the WD-repeat containing domains, that are assembled into trimers by virtue of the presence of the C-terminal coiled coil domain.[8]

The assembly of the coiled coil domain into trimers, rather than the previously assumed dimer was further confirmed by X-ray crystallography.[21] Interestingly, it turned out that the coronin 1

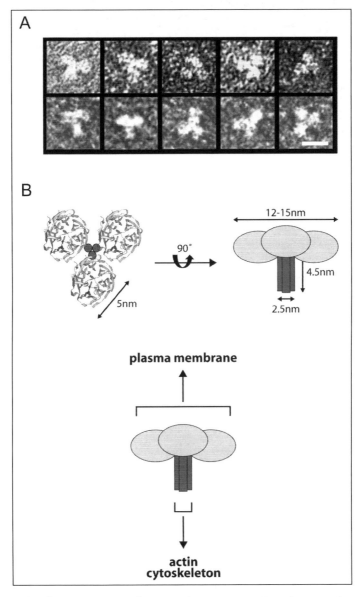

Figure 2. Molecular organization of coronin 1. A) Transmission electron micrographs of affinity-purified and negatively stained coronin 1 (coronin 1A) complexes isolated from macrophages. The gallery shows multiple examples of the trimeric structure. Scale bar, 10 nm. From.[8] B) Cartoon presenting the organization of the coronin 1 trimer deduced from the image analysis.

coiled coil contains a distinct structural motif, encompassing specific networks of surface salt bridges that is conserved among a variety of trimeric coiled coils.[21] In this light it will be interesting to analyze the biophysical and biochemical characteristics of the coiled coil domains from other coronin isoforms.

Function of Coronin 1 in Leukocytes

Coronin 1 (coronin 1A), in contrast to several ubiquitously expressed coronin isoforms, is exclusively expressed in leukocytes.[3] Thus far, coronin 1 expression has been demonstrated in thymocytes, T-cells, macrophages and neutrophils.[2,3,22-24] Morphological examination of coronin 1 in thymocytes and T-cells shows its accumulation at sites of membrane activity and actin rearrangement.[22,23] It has recently been suggested that in T-cells, coronin 1 prevents F-actin induced apoptosis.[23] However, in coronin 1 deficient mice all other leukocyte populations are present in normal numbers, arguing against a general role for coronin 1 in preventing apoptosis.

Coronin 1 in Macrophages

One of the first reports on a role for coronin 1 in leukocytes implicated coronin 1 in the intracellular survival of pathogenic mycobacteria.[3] While most other bacteria upon internalization in macrophages are rapidly transferred from phagosomes to lysosomes followed by their destruction, mycobacteria, once internalized, actively block the fusion of phagosomes with lysosomes.[25-27]

A search for host molecules possibly involved in mediating the block in phagosome-lysosome fusion, identified coronin 1 (then known as TACO, for Tryptophan Aspartate containing Coat protein) as the sole detectable protein exclusively retained on mycobacterial phagosomes.[3] Coronin 1, which in non-infected macrophages distributes equally between the cytosol and the membranes, is exclusively retained on phagosomes of macrophages infected with live mycobacteria, whereas in macrophages infected with dead mycobacteria, coronin 1 is initially co-internalized but rapidly dissociates from phagosomes. Following dissociation, the noncoated phagosomes fuse with or mature into lysosomes, resulting in the subsequent degradation of the internalized mycobacteria. This suggested an essential role for coronin 1 in preventing the fusion of mycobacterial phagosomes with lysosomes.[3,28] Moreover, mycobacteria are effectively destroyed within Kupffer cells, the resident macrophages of the liver that do not express coronin 1.[3] Interestingly, virulent strains of the human pathogen *H. pylori* are equally capable to actively retain coronin 1 at the phagosomal membrane upon internalization, suggesting that the coronin 1-mediated block in lysosomal fusion might be utilized also by other pathogens.[29] However, whether or not pathogen specific molecules are involved in the active phagosomal retention of coronin 1 remains is as yet unclear.

How coronin 1 mediates the survival of pathogenic mycobacteria has remained obscure. While a direct contribution of coronin 1 to the internalization of mycobacteria could be excluded early on, its molecular role remained enigmatic. The analysis of a genetic model for coronin 1, however, has recently shed some light on the molecular activities of coronin 1 in macrophages. It turned out that, while being fully dispensible for all F-actin-mediated functions analyzed (phagocytosis, macropinocytosis, motility), coronin 1 is required for the activation of the Ca^{2+} dependent phosphatase calcineurin.[30] In wild type macrophages, upon internalization of mycobacteria this phosphatase becomes activated, thereby blocking phagosome-lysosome fusion by an as yet unknown mechanism and allowing mycobacterial survival (see also Fig. 3). In the absence of coronin 1, calcineurin activation does not occur resulting in phagosome-lysosome fusion and intracellular killing of the internalized mycobacteria. Strikingly, the genetic depletion of coronin 1 can be phenocopied by the addition of the calcineurin inhibitors cyclosporin A and FK506. Thus, it appears that coronin 1 has evolved to activate Ca^{2+} dependent signaling reactions in macrophages thereby promoting the survival of pathogenic mycobacteria.[30] How, exactly, coronin 1 mediates the activation of calcineurin remains to be analyzed and may be related to its activity in modulating the association of membranes with the cytoskeleton.[8]

A role for coronin 1 in the regulation of signaling reactions in leukocytes is also consistent with its localization within cholesterol-enriched domains[31,32] as well as to a possible role for protein kinase

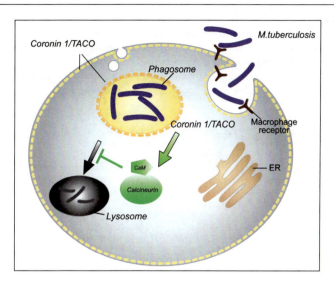

Figure 3. Model for the Activity of Coronin 1 in Macrophages. In resting macrophages, coronin 1 (coronin 1A) is distributed between the cytoplasm as well as the cell cortex. Upon the entry of pathogenic mycobacteria, coronin 1 is recruited and actively retained at the phagosomal membrane, thereby ensuring the activation of calcineurin. Activation of calcineurin results in a block in the fusion of mycobacterial phagosomes with lysosomes. As a consequence, deletion of coronin 1 or inhibiting calcineurin activity results in the induction of phagosome lysosome fusion and mycobacterial killing.

C in the modulation of its localization.[33,34] Cholesterol-enriched domains are known to harbor a subset of molecules involved in signaling.[35-37] Since in the absence of cholesterol mycobacteria are not even phagocytosed,[31,38] it is well possible that mycobacteria have evolved mechanisms that ensure their uptake in a cholesterol dependent manner such that once they are internalized, they can reside within coronin 1-coated phagosomes. Consequently, the recruited coronin 1 then activates calcineurin resulting in blocking phagolysosome fusion and preventing degradation of the bacilli, thereby allowing the mycobacteria to survive intracellularly (Fig. 3).

Importantly, corroborating the original observation that coronin 1 was not involved in mycobacterial uptake, macrophages devoid of coronin 1 were perfectly capable to internalize mycobacteria as well as a range of other phagocytic cargo.[30] Thus, in contrast to the situation in *Dictyostelium*, coronin 1 is dispensable for phagocytosis in macrophages. Also, several other actin-dependent processes, such as macropinocytosis, cell motility, cell spreading and membrane ruffling were unaffected in macrophages lacking coronin. These results strongly suggest that in macrophages, coronin 1 is dispensable for F-actin mediated processes.

Conclusions and Perspectives

Coronin 1 (coronin 1A) is probably one of the best-characterized members of the coronin protein family expressed in vertebrates. Emerging evidence suggests that, at least in macrophages, rather than being involved in F-actin mediated processes, coronin 1 modulates the activation of signaling reactions. In doing so, the presence or absence of coronin 1 regulates the intracellular trafficking as well as the survival of pathogenic mycobacteria. Since macrophages lacking coronin 1 are fully functional, the role for coronin 1 in uninfected cells remains enigmatic. The availability of different model systems is however likely to allow the dissection of the true role of this abundant molecule not only in macrophages but also in other leukocyte subpopulations.

Acknowledgement

I thank the members of my laboratory for many stimulating discussions, Benoit Combulazier, Rajesh Jayachandran, Philipp Mueller and Varadha Sundaramurthy for critical reading of the manuscript and Annette Roulier for assistance in the artwork. Research in my laboratory is supported by the Swiss National Science Foundation, the Roche Research Foundation, the Olga Mayenfisch Foundations as well as the Swiss Lung Liga and the Swiss Life Jubileum Stiftung.

References

1. de Hostos EL, Bradtke B, Lottspeich F et al. Coronin, an actin binding protein of Dictyostelium discoideum localized to cell surface projections, has sequence similarities to G protein beta subunits. EMBO J 1991; 10(13):4097-4104.
2. Suzuki K, Nishihata J, Arai Y et al. Molecular cloning of a novel actin-binding protein, p57, with a WD repeat and a leucine zipper motif. FEBS Lett 1995; 364(3):283-288.
3. Ferrari G, Langen H, Naito M et al. A coat protein on phagosomes involved in the intracellular survival of mycobacteria. Cell 1999; 97(4):435-447.
4. Heil-Chapdelaine RA, Tran NK, Cooper JA. The role of Saccharomyces cerevisiae coronin in the actin and microtubule cytoskeletons. Curr Biol 1998; 8(23):1281-1284.
5. Humphries CL, Balcer HI, D'Agostino JL et al. Direct regulation of Arp2/3 complex activity and function by the actin binding protein coronin. J Cell Biol 2002; 159(6):993-1004.
6. Rappleye CA, Paredez AR, Smith CW et al. The coronin-like protein POD-1 is required for anterior-posterior axis formation and cellular architecture in the nematode caenorhabditis elegans. Genes Dev 1999; 13(21):2838-2851.
7. Rothenberg ME, Rogers SL, Vale RD et al. Drosophila pod-1 crosslinks both actin and microtubules and controls the targeting of axons. Neuron 2003; 39(5):779-791.
8. Gatfield J, Albrecht I, Zanolari B et al. Association of the Leukocyte Plasma Membrane with the Actin Cytoskeleton through Coiled Coil-mediated Trimeric Coronin 1 Molecules. Mol Biol Cell 2005; 16(6):2786-2798.
9. de Hostos EL. The coronin family of actin-associated proteins. Trends Cell Biol 1999; 9(9):345-350.
10. van der Voorn L, Ploegh HL. The WD-40 repeat. FEBS Lett 1992; 307(2):131-134.
11. Simon MI, Strathmann MP, Gautam N. Diversity of G proteins in signal transduction. Science 1991; 252(5007):802-808.
12. Neer EJ, Schmidt CJ, Nambudripad R et al. The ancient regulatory-protein family of WD-repeat proteins. Nature 1994; 371(6495):297-300.
13. Li D, Roberts R. WD-repeat proteins: structure characteristics, biological function and their involvement in human diseases. Cell Mol Life Sci 2001; 58(14):2085-2097.
14. Yu L, Gaitatzes C, Neer E et al. Thirty-plus functional families from a single motif. Protein Sci 2000; 9(12):2470-2476.
15. Fulop V, Jones DT. Beta propellers: structural rigidity and functional diversity. Curr Opin Struct Biol 1999; 9(6):715-721.
16. Smith TF, Gaitatzes C, Saxena K et al. The WD repeat: a common architecture for diverse functions. Trends Biochem Sci 1999; 24(5):181-185.
17. Jawad Z, Paoli M. Novel sequences propel familiar folds. Structure (Camb) 2002; 10(4):447-454.
18. Appleton BA, Wu P, Wiesmann C. The crystal structure of murine coronin-1: a regulator of actin cytoskeletal dynamics in lymphocytes. Structure 2006; 14(1):87-96.
19. Sprague ER, Redd MJ, Johnson AD et al. Structure of the C-terminal domain of Tup1, a corepressor of transcription in yeast. EMBO J 2000; 19(12):3016-3027.
20. Lambright DG, Sondek J, Bohm A et al. The 2.0 A crystal structure of a heterotrimeric G protein. Nature 1996; 379(6563):311-319.
21. Kammerer RA, Kostrewa D, Progias P et al. A conserved trimerization motif controls the topology of short coiled coils. Proc Natl Acad Sci USA 2005; 102(39):13891-13896.
22. Nal B, Carroll P, Mohr E et al. Coronin-1 expression in T-lymphocytes: insights into protein function during T-cell development and activation. Int Immunol 2004; 16(2):231-240.
23. Foger N, Rangell L, Danilenko DM et al. Requirement for coronin 1 in T-lymphocyte trafficking and cellular homeostasis. Science 2006; 313(5788):839-842.
24. Grogan A, Reeves E, Keep N et al. Cytosolic phox proteins interact with and regulate the assembly of coronin in neutrophils. J Cell Sci 1997; 110(Pt 24):3071-3081.
25. Armstrong JA, Hart DPA. Response of cultured macrophages to Mycobacterium tuberculosis, with observations on fusion of lysosomes with phagosomes. J Exp Med 1971; 134:713-740.
26. Russell DG. Mycobacterium tuberculosis: here today and here tomorrow. Nat Rev Mol Cell Biol 2001; 2(8):569-577.

27. Pieters J. Manipulation of the Macrophage Response by Pathogenic Mycobacteria. In: Kaufmann Sea, Rubin E, eds. Handbook of Tuberculosis: Molecular Biology and Biochemistry: Wiley-VCH; 2007.
28. Tailleux L, Neyrolles O, Honore-Bouakline S et al. Constrained intracellular survival of Mycobacterium tuberculosis in human dendritic cells. J Immunol 2003; 170(4):1939-1948.
29. Zheng PY, Jones NL. Helicobacter pylori strains expressing the vacuolating cytotoxin interrupt phagosome maturation in macrophages by recruiting and retaining TACO (coronin 1) protein. Cell Microbiol 2003; 5(1):25-40.
30. Jayachandran R, Sundaramurthy V, Combaluzier B et al. Survival of mycobacteria in macrophages is mediated by coronin 1-dependent activation of calcineurin. Cell 2007; 130(1):37-50.
31. Gatfield J, Pieters J. Essential role for cholesterol in entry of mycobacteria into macrophages. Science 2000; 288(5471):1647-1650.
32. Pieters J, Gatfield J. Hijacking the host: survival of pathogenic mycobacteria inside macrophages. Trends Microbiol 2002; 10(3):142-146.
33. Itoh S, Suzuki K, Nishihata J et al. The role of protein kinase C in the transient association of p57, a coronin family actin-binding protein, with phagosomes. Biol Pharm Bull 2002; 25(7):837-844.
34. Reeves EP, Dekker LV, Forbes LV et al. Direct interaction between p47phox and protein kinase C: evidence for targeting of protein kinase C by p47phox in neutrophils. Biochem J 1999; 344 (Pt 3):859-866.
35. Brown DA, London E. Structure and function of sphingolipid- and cholesterol-rich membrane rafts. J Biol Chem 2000; 275(23):17221-17224.
36. Simons K, Ikonen E. Functional rafts in cell membranes. Nature 1997; 387(6633):569-572.
37. Kaul D, Anand PK, Verma I. Cholesterol-sensor initiates M. tuberculosis entry into human macrophages. Mol Cell Biochem 2004; 258(1-2):219-222.
38. Peyron P, Bordier C, N'Diaye EN et al. Nonopsonic phagocytosis of Mycobacterium kansasii by human neutrophils depends on cholesterol and is mediated by CR3 associated with glycosylphosphatidylinositol-anchored proteins. J Immunol 2000; 165(9):5186-5191.

CHAPTER 11

The Role of Mammalian Coronins in Development and Disease

David W. Roadcap, Christoph S. Clemen[†] and James E. Bear[†*]

Abstract

Coronins have maintained a high degree of conservation over the roughly 800 million years of eukaryotic evolution.[1,2] From its origins as a single gene in simpler eukaryotes, the mammalian Coronin gene family has expanded to include at least six members (see Chapter 4). Increasing evidence indicates that Coronins play critical roles as regulators of actin dependent processes such as cell motility and vesicle trafficking[3,4] (see Chapters 6-9). Considering the importance of these processes, it is not surprising that recent findings have implicated the involvement of Coronins in multiple diseases. This review primarily focuses on Coronin 1C (HGNC symbol: CORO1C, also known as Coronin 3) which is a transcriptionally dynamic gene that is up-regulated in multiple types of clinically aggressive cancer. In addition to reviewing the molecular signals and events that lead to Coronin 1C transcription, we summarize the results of several studies describing the possible functional roles of Coronin 1C in development as well as disease progression. Here, the main focus is on brain development and on the progression of melanoma and glioma. Finally, we will also review the role of other mammalian Coronin genes in clinically relevant processes such as neural regeneration and pathogenic bacterial infections (see Chapter 10).

Coronin 1C: A Transcriptionally Dynamic Coronin Gene

One member of the mammalian Coronin gene family that is frequently observed to be up- or down-regulated in DNA microarray experiments is Coronin 1C. These data strongly suggest that this gene is transcriptionally dynamic, a finding supported by the fact that Coronin 1C was discovered in the early '90s as a gene that is induced by serum stimulation in fibroblasts.[5] In this early work, Coronin 1C was identified as mig-3 for mitogen induced gene 3 and was not pursued. In 2004, Coronin 1C was independently identified as a serum-induced gene as part of a systematic search for genes that reflected a 'wound signature' in fibroblasts.[6] The authors reasoned that fibroblast wound healing and tumor metastasis likely share a common set of up-regulated genes that may have prognostic value for clinical outcomes. Indeed, the expression of the 512 genes identified as part of the 'core serum response' does have strong predictive value for patient survival across a variety of tumors. More recently, Coronin 1C was identified as a delayed primary response gene in PDGF-stimulated glioblastoma cells.[7] Together, these studies demonstrate that Coronin 1C is up-regulated at the transcriptional level by extracellular stimuli such as serum and growth factors. However, since these stimuli activate a large number of signaling cascades, these studies do not reveal much about the specific molecular events that increase Coronin 1C transcription.

[†]These authors contributed equally to this work.
*Corresponding Author: James E. Bear—UNC-Chapel Hill, Lineberger Comprehensive Cancer Center and Department of Cell and Developmental Biology, CB #7295, Chapel Hill, NC 27599, USA. Email: jbear@email.unc.edu

The Coronin Family of Proteins, edited by Christoph S. Clemen, Ludwig Eichinger and Vasily Rybakin. ©2008 Landes Bioscience and Springer Science+Business Media.

In addition to these studies, other experiments have identified Coronin 1C as a target of specific pathways utilizing the transcription factors c-Myc/Max and Slug/Snail/E47. The activity of c-Myc and its partner Max has been frequently associated with human malignancies by contributing to cellular transformation and evasion of apoptosis. Coronin 1C was identified in a genome wide screen for promoters that bound to c-Myc in Burkitt's lymphoma cells.[8] While this finding is intriguing, it is worth noting that this screen yielded a large number of target genes (>900) and may reflect global transcriptional regulation by c-Myc. In a more specific screen, Coronin 1C was identified as one of twenty target genes that were up-regulated upon expression of the transcription factors Snail, Slug and E47 in epithelial cells.[9] Each of these transcription factors has been associated with epithelial-to-mesenchymal transition (EMT) in epithelial cells and they are consistently over-expressed in carcinoma cell lines with invasive and metastatic properties. This result suggests that Coronin 1C may be a strong candidate as both a biomarker for invasive cancer and functionally important for disease progression.

Consistent with the transcriptional dynamism of Coronin 1C, many other studies have identified this gene as either up- or down-regulated under various conditions (Fig. 1 and Table 1) and here we will highlight several of these studies that relate to cancer progression. Endometrial carcinoma (EC) is an extremely common gynecological malignancy that comprises two different types of tumor with a more benign type I EC and the more clinically aggressive nonendometrioid endometrial carcinoma (NEEC). Coronin 1C is up-regulated 2.3 fold in NEEC relative to type I EC.[10] In another study, Coronin 1C was identified as part of a 99-gene hypoxia expression signature in head and neck squamous cell carcinomas (HNSCC).[11] Since hypoxia is a strong negative prognostic factor in many tumors including HNSCC, this also points to the involvement of Coronin 1C in disease progression in this malignancy.[12] Finally, Coronin 1C was identified as one of 79 genes up-regulated in androgen-insensitive prostate cancer cell lines relative to androgen-sensitive cell lines.[13] Since androgen insensitivity is a hallmark of aggressive prostate cancer, this further reinforces the link between Coronin 1C expression and invasion and metastasis.[14]

Coronin 1C as a Marker of Melanoma Progression

Advanced melanoma is one of the most feared human cancers.[15,16] Although curable through surgery when diagnosed at early stage, melanoma is characterized by its therapeutic resistance and aggressive clinical behavior. A proclivity for early metastasis is a key clinical feature of melanoma and in perhaps no other malignancy is the ability to metastasize more closely correlated with clinical outcome.[17,18] On the molecular level, one of the signature genetic events of melanoma is activation of the Ras/Raf pathway, with the majority (90%) of human melanomas harboring activating mutations in either N-RAS or B-RAF.[19-21] Activation of either of these molecules induces persistent activation of the Erk mitogen-activated protein kinase (MAPK) cascade,[22] suggesting that aberrant activation of the Erk pathway is a critical step in melanoma development. A major consequence of Erk activation is regulation of gene expression. However, the gene targets of this

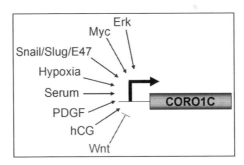

Figure 1. Inputs into the Coronin 1C promoter. Schematic diagram of the known signaling inputs that affect Coronin 1C transcription.

Table 1. Conditions under which Coronin 1C is transcriptionally regulated

Stimulus	Coro1C Expression	Reference
ERK	Up	26
PDGF	Up	7
Hypoxia	Up	11
Human Respiratory Syncytial Virus Infection	Up	61
Wnt	Down	62
Adenovirus	Down	63
Snail, Slug and E47	Up	9
Myelodysplastic syndrome Development	Up	64
Androgen Sensitive vs Insensitive Prostate Cancer	Insensitive higher	13
Serum	Up	5,6
Gefitinib Responsive vs Unresponsive Patients	Unresponsive higher	65
Cytomegalovirus Infection	Down	66
Chronic Obstructive Pulmonary disease Progression	Down	67
Fibronectin-Induced Cardiomyocye Hypertrophy	Up	68
Nonendometriod Carcinomas	Up	10
Myc and Max	Up	8
Dendritic Cell Maturation	Down	69
Acute Lymphatic Leukemia	Up	70

pathway important for oncogenesis in melanoma have only recently begun to be elucidated.[23] These gene expression experiments and those from other groups have shown that cytoskeletal regulatory genes are frequently up-regulated during metastasis,[24,25] highlighting the importance of cell migration in the etiology of metastatic cancer. Understanding how actin dynamics become mis-regulated during metastasis may allow the identification of new diagnostic markers that predict metastatic potential and provide candidate targets for clinical intervention.

Recent work has examined Coronin 1C protein levels in both normal human skin and human melanoma.[26] Immunohistochemical staining reveals that, in normal skin, Coronin 1C levels are relatively low (Fig. 2A). This starkly contrasts with severe dysplastic nevi (abnormal moles more likely to develop into melanomas) and metastases, where the staining of tumor cells is much stronger (Fig. 2A). In order to determine if Erk is responsible for Coronin 1C up-regulation, three B-RAF mutant melanoma cell lines with high phospho-Erk levels (WM2664, SKMel24 and SKMel28) were examined by quantitative real-time PCR.[23] All three contain high levels of Coronin 1C mRNA which are significantly reduced upon treatment with the Erk inhibitor U0126 (Fig. 2B). These data indicate that Coronin 1C is a potential marker for melanoma progression and that its expression is at least partly dependent on activation of the Erk pathway.

Coronin 1C Expression Is Regulated during Murine Brain Development

The dynamics of Coronin 1C (Coronin 3) expression have also been studied in both the development and diseased state of the brain. Studies of Coronin 1C in brain tumor cells revealed a similar story to that presented above for melanoma and are presented in the next section of this chapter. Coronin 1C expression was also high in all regions of the developing brain and this section discusses the developmental and cell specific expression patterns that are observed during further brain maturation.[27]

The neocortex consists of different laminae that are formed sequentially during the first postnatal days with the inner laminae differentiating first.[28] Coronin 1C expression follows this inside-out gradient and deeper cortical layers are the first to show a decrease in the expression of Coronin 1C.

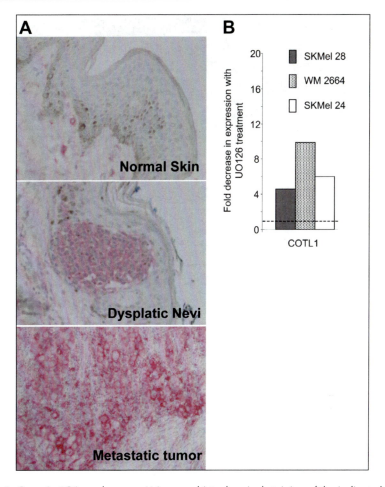

Figure 2. Coronin 1C in melanoma. A) Immunohistochemical staining of the indicated tissue samples for Coronin 1C. 5 μm sections from melanoma tumors were stained with a new Coronin 1C specific mAb (Roadcap and Bear, unpublished reagent) for 30min at 37°C with a steam heat-induced epitope retrieval, using the streptavidin/biotin method with an alkaline phosphatase label and Permanent Red (Dako) as the chromogen and then stained with hematoxylin. B) qRT-PCR analysis of the indicated melanoma cell lines treated with the Erk inhibitor U0126 or vehicle control for 24 hours.[26] Dotted line indicates 1x threshold.

By the later stages of brain development, Coronin 1C is detected only in a small peripheral cortical layer. Finally, only weak basal levels of Coronin 1C remain detectable after terminal differentiation of the cortical neurons (Fig. 3A, P1 and P20 are shown). Similarly, the high levels of Coronin 1C in immature neurons of the cerebellum are decreased after formation of the granule cell layers (Fig. 3B). Some types of neurons, including hippocampal pyramidal CA1-CA3 and Purkinje cells, retain strong expression of Coronin 1C until early murine adulthood (Fig. 3C, left image, analyzed up to 80 days). These neurons harbor a high degree of synaptic plasticity, which enables them to undergo long-term potentiation and depression processes like learning and memory.[29-32] Inversely to the patterns of the grey matter, areas of the white matter increase the expression of Coronin 1C (Fig. 3C, right image, only P30 is shown) during the progress of myelination.[33,34] It has been suggested that these localization patterns place Coronin 1C in a position to play a role in diverse

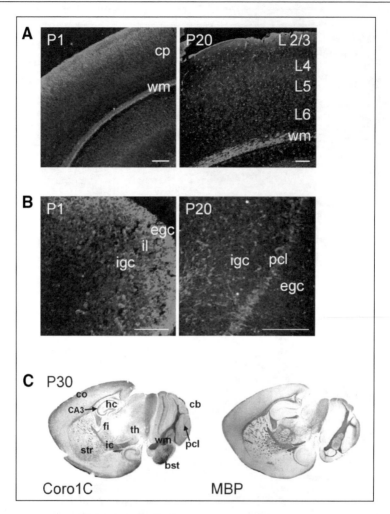

Figure 3. Coronin 1C expression levels during maturation of the grey and white matter of murine brain. Localization of Coronin 1C (Coronin 3) in sections of postnatal neocortex (A) and cerebellar sections (B, one folium is shown) of stages P1 and P20 analyzed by immunofluorescence. Coronal 6 μm sections from paraffin-embedded brains were stained with Coronin 1C specific mAb K6-444. Cp, cortical plate; L1-L6, cortical layers; wm, white matter; egc, external granule cell layer; igc, internal granule cell layer; il, intermediate layer; pcl, Purkinje cell layer. Bars, 200 μm (A), 100 μm (B). C) Distribution of Coronin 1C and myelin basic protein in total brains from postnatal day 30 analyzed by mAb K6-444 (left image) or rat monoclonal anti-MBP (right image) and visualized by DAB staining. Bst, brain stem; cb, cerebellum; co, neocortex; fi, fimbria; hc, hippocampus; ic, internal capsule; str, striatum; th, thalamus; wm, white matter of the cerebellum; pcl, Purkinje cell layer; CA3, hippocampal pyramidal CA3. Bar, 1 mm. Images according to Hasse et al (2005).[27]

processes such as neuronal migration, differentiation, formation of neurites and the formation of lamellar protrusions and myelin sheaths of oligodendroglial cells.[27]

These tightly controlled expression patterns suggest that imbalances in the expression of Coronin 1C during brain development might lead to defects in brain morphology. This hypothesis is supported by the observation that another member of the Coronin protein family, Coronin

1A, exhibits reduced expression levels in Down syndrome brain.[35] It is noteworthy that other WD40-repeat containing proteins—Coronin proteins represent the cytoskeleton-related subfamily of WD40-repeat proteins (see Chapter 2)—also have been linked to human diseases with malformations of the nervous system, namely the lissencephaly,[36,37] Cockayne syndrome,[38] late-onset sensorineural deafness[39] and the alacrima-achalasia-adrenal insufficiency (triple-A-syndrome).[40,41]

Coronin 1C Is Associated with the Malignant Phenotype of Human Diffuse Gliomas

In parallel to the work on Coronin 1C (Coronin 3) in melanoma progression, Coronin 1C's role in coordinating migration and invasion of tumor cells in the human brain has been investigated. Previously, Coronin 1C was reported to exert a role in regulation of F-actin turnover during cell migration and neurite outgrowth.[4,42] To address a possible role of Coronin 1C in brain tumor cells, its expression in normal human brain tissue and various entities of human brain tumors was determined.[43]

In the normal adult human brain tissue, neurons in the cortex have little Coronin 1C, while the white matter do not show any significant expression. In brain tumors, the expression levels of Coronin 1C depend on the tumor type. Benign meningiomas (Fig. 4A, left image), pilocytic astrocytomas, high-grade anaplastic astrocytomas, oligodendrogliomas, oligoastrocytomas and glioblastomas all strongly express Coronin 1C. Low grade diffuse astrocytomas (Fig. 4A, right image), oligodendrogliomas and oligoastrocytomas show only weak staining of Coronin 1C in the tumor cells, while no expression of Coronin 1C is detectable in tumors of neuronal origin like the desmoplastic medulloblastoma and neuroblastoma. In mixed glial tumors, the astroglial portion of the tumor often expresses Coronin 1C at higher levels than the oligodendroglial component. Within an individual tumor, tumor cells adjacent to proliferating microvessels exhibit a stronger Coronin 1C staining than those adjacent to areas of necrosis (Fig. 4B). In addition, the tumor matrix contains a varying number of reactive astrocytes, activated and migrating astrocytic cells, which also highly express Coronin 1C. This also was the case for reactive astrocytes and microglial cells that had been triggered by circumscriptive nontumor lesions such as infarcts and traumatic lesions (Fig. 4C, left image). In contrast, reactive astrocytes in epilepsia-related diffuse astrogliosis less strongly express Coronin 1C.

A finding of significance is that Coronin 1C was associated with the malignant phenotype of diffuse gliomas.[43] This class of tumors includes astrocytomas, oligodendrogliomas and oligoastrocytomas. Diffuse gliomas clearly have a strong correlation between high Coronin 1C expression levels and increased grade of the malignancy (Fig. 4C, right image). Coronin 1C's demonstrated role in actin dynamics and cell motility suggests that its expression in astroglial cells and in glial tumor cells is related to migration and the malignant phenotype. This hypothesis was tested by shRNA-mediated knockdown of Coronin 1C in U373 and A172 glioblastoma cells.[43] Silencing Coronin 1C expression significantly reduces cell proliferation rates, cell migration velocity, formation of invadopodia, secretion of matrix metalloproteinases and invasion into extracellular matrix (Fig. 5A-C and data not shown). Previously, the degree of migration and invasion of tumor cells into healthy tissue was found to be a critical parameter of malignancy in diffuse gliomas and, moreover, a factor that limits the success of surgery.[44] Thus, these data provide strong evidence that the expression level of Coronin 1C correlates with the grade of malignancy of diffuse gliomas and that Coronin 1C is significantly involved in tumor cell proliferation, migration, invasion, malignant progression and possibly prognosis of diffuse gliomas.

Other Coronin Genes and Disease

Coronin 1A (Coronin 1) is highly expressed in the hematopoetic system and regulates F-actin content in thymocytes (discussed below).[45] Gene expression array studies suggest that its expression may be altered in lymphomas and other tumors of hematopoetic origin, although there is no apparent trend between cancer progression and Coronin 1A expression.[46-50] Since control of actin dynamics is an integral part many disease states, it follows that Coronins could play a role in

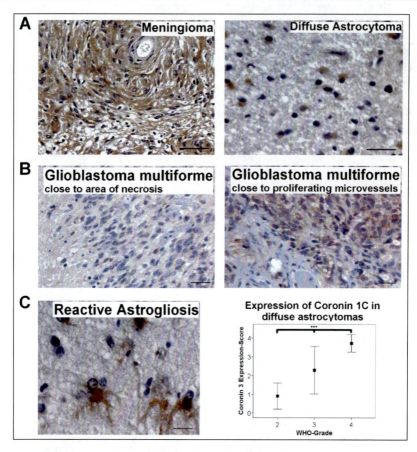

Figure 4. Coronin 1C expression levels are associated with the malignant phenotype of human gliomas. Paraffin-embedded tissue sections of human brain tumors were immunostained with a monoclonal antibody directed against Coronin 1C (Coronin 3), followed by biotinylated secondary antibodies and the avidin-peroxidase complex with 3,3-diaminobencidine as substrate. A) Coronin 1C is widely expressed in the benign meningotheliomatous meningioma (WHO-grade I), bar, 70 μm; the diffuse astrocytoma (a low grade diffuse glioma) showed Coronin 1C expression in no more than 50% of the tumors cells, bar, 25 μm. B) In a glioblastoma multiforme nearly all tumor cells expressed Coronin 1C, the most prominent expression was detected in areas of vital tumor with microvascular proliferation while surviving tumor cells near areas of palisading necroses were only weakly labeled; bars, 40 μm. (C, left image) Activated astrocytes strongly exhibiting Coronin 1C were present in the brain close to an infarct lesion in the stage of beginning gliosis; bar, 10 μm. (C, right image) Tumor cell expression in relation to malignancy was determined by quantification of the immunohistochemical expression of Coronin 1C in diffuse gliomas. With increasing malignancy as indicated by the WHO-grade the expression of Coronin 1C in diffuse gliomas increased. Mean and standard deviation are presented; ***indicates $p < 0.01$ as calculated by the Kruskal-Wallis H-test and the trend-test. Images according to Thal et al.[43]

diseases other than cancer. The best-characterized example of this is Coronin 1A's role in pathogenic bacterial infection.[51] The standard immune response to bacterial infection involves macrophages engulfing bacteria via phagocytosis. By utilizing controlled membrane fusion of phagosomes with lysosomes, the macrophages are able to deliver lytic enzymes, acidify phagolysosomes and

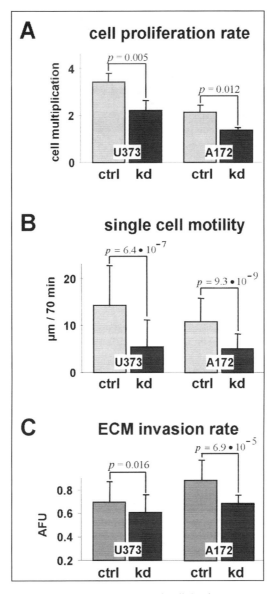

Figure 5. Coronin 1C influences malignancy-related cellular functions. A) Proliferation rates of U373 and A172 glioblastoma cells lacking Coronin 1C (Coronin 3) expression (kd) are compared to control cells (ctrl); a certain number of cells was seeded and counted again after two days; four independent experiments each, Student's t-test; U373: factor 2.2 vs. 3.4, p = 0.005; A172: factor 1.4 vs 2.1, p = 0.012. B) Coronin 1C knockdown reduced the motility of single cells; the chart indicates the values from a total of 40 cells derived from several independent experiments; Student's t-test; U373: velocity 5.36 μm/70min vs. 14.3 μm/70min, p = 6.4×10^{-7}; A172: velocity 5.0 μm/70min vs 10.9 μm/70min, p = 9.3×10^{-9}. C) Invasion of U373 and A172 glioblastoma cells lacking Coronin 1C expression into extracellular matrix; a representative experiment with mean and standard deviation of 40 and 20 measurements of U373 and A172 glioblastoma cells, respectively; Student's t-test; U373: 0.6 AFU vs. 0.7 AFU, p = 0.016; A172: 0.7 AFU vs. 0.9 AFU, p = 6.9×10^{-5}. Images according to Thal et al.[43]

subsequently destroy the bacteria.[52] Nucleation of actin filaments around nascent phagosomes plays an important role in mediating these critical vesicle fusion events and thus the immune response to bacterial infection can be considered an actin-dependent process.[53] Pathogenic bacteria such as *Mycobacterium tuberculosis* can circumvent the response by retaining Coronin 1A (called TACO in the original study) on the phagosome surface, thereby preventing the maturation of the phagosomes and allowing bacterial propagation within the macrophage.[51] The mechanism of retention of Coronin 1A on bacterial-containing phagosomes was unclear for many years. A recent study, however, has identified the bacterial protein lipoamide dehydrogenase C (LpdC) as a Coronin 1A binding protein that recruits and retains Coronin 1A on the phagosome.[54] In this work, the authors demonstrated that enforced expression of LpdC increased the survival of normally nonpathogenic bacteria in macrophages. Together, these data are highly suggestive that pathogenic bacteria are hijacking Coronin 1A function to alter actin dynamics on macrophage phagosomes and thereby evading the normal immune response.

Alternately, evidence also exists that Coronin 1A's role may be to control calcium dynamics after bacterial infection.[55] Macrophages from mice lacking Coronin 1A do not display the persistent increase in calcium levels that are normally displayed after infection. This consequently prevents the activation of signaling pathways via proteins such as the calcium-sensitive phosphatase Calcineurin. While no alterations in actin dependent processes have been detected in Coronin 1A null macrophages, the effects may be linked to more subtle effects on actin that affect the known relationship between cytoskeletal dynamics and calcium trafficking.[56,57] Dramatic effects on actin-dependent processes may also be masked by the presence of functionally redundant Coronin isoforms in this cell type.

While Coronin 1A is utilized to the detriment of macrophages after pathogenic bacterial infection, it plays a large role in the normal immune system as the most prominent hematopoietic Coronin.[45] For instance, T-cells from Coronin 1A null mice are profoundly defective in both their ability to undergo chemotaxis in vitro and to home to secondary lymphocyte organs in vivo. Together, these defects lead to a decrease in the levels of CD4$^+$ and CD8$^+$ T-cells in the blood, spleen and lymph nodes of Coronin 1A deficient mice. This phenotype was linked to Coronin 1A's ability to control steady-state F-actin levels via regulation of Arp2/3. Loss of Coronin 1A could therefore lead to an increased rate of immune system failure and a consequent susceptibility to numerous diseases, although this hypothesis has yet to be tested. Further information on Coronin proteins in lymphocytes and macrophages can be found in Chapters 8 6th section and 10.

Coronin 1B (Coronin 2) is the most ubiquitously expressed mammalian isoform of Coronin, but relatively few studies have examined its role in disease states.[58] It has, however, been linked to neurite formation and axon regeneration following spinal cord injury.[59] p53 activation following injury stimulates the formation and growth of neurites that facilitate regeneration of neural pathways and knockdown of Coronin 1B decreases this neurite outgrowth.[60] Coronin 1B activity therefore, like that of Coronin 1C, may be linked to neurodegenerative diseases or even control of neuronal plasticity. Further study of Coronin 1B is necessary to facilitate understanding of its role in diseases, but there is strong evidence that it plays an important role in regulating actin dynamics at the leading edge of motile cells.[3] Disruption of this process may be important for a number of motility-involving diseases.

Unanswered Questions and Future Directions

Although Coronins (and particularly Coronin 1C (Coronin 3)) have been implicated in disease states, much work remains to establish functional links between transcriptional regulation and phenotypic change. One important area that will require more work is the careful delineation of the Coronin 1C promoter and its immediate upstream inputs. In addition, the biochemical mechanism of Coronin 1C activity needs to be more precisely determined and the relevant binding partners necessary for this activity need to be identified. Understanding these issues may be important for revealing how diverse signaling cascades are dis-regulated in invasive/metastatic cancer. Another area that will require future studies is clarifying the role that Coronin proteins play in development. Continued analysis of mouse gene deletion models should be quite informative in this regard.

Acknowledgements

We would like to thank Dan Zedek, Nancy Thomas and Nick Holoweckyj for contributions to Figure 2. DR is supported by NIH (NRSA, F32 CA128297), CSC is supported by the DFG (NO 113/13-3) and Köln Fortune, JEB is supported by the Melanoma Research Foundation and the Sontag Foundation.

References

1. Rybakin V, Clemen CS. Coronin proteins as multifunctional regulators of the cytoskeleton and membrane trafficking. Bioessays 2005; 27(6):625-632.
2. Uetrecht AC, Bear JE. Coronins: the return of the crown. Trends Cell Biol 2006; 16(8):421-426.
3. Cai L, Marshall TW, Uetrecht AC et al. Coronin 1B coordinates Arp2/3 complex and cofilin activities at the leading edge. Cell 2007; 128(5):915-929.
4. Rosentreter A, Hofmann A, Xavier CP et al. Coronin 3 involvement in F-actin-dependent processes at the cell cortex. Exp Cell Res 2007; 313(5):878-895.
5. Wick M, Burger C, Brusselbach S et al. Identification of serum-inducible genes: different patterns of gene regulation during G0—>S and G1—>S progression. J Cell Sci 1994; 107 (Pt 1):227-239.
6. Chang HY, Sneddon JB, Alizadeh AA et al. Gene Expression Signature of Fibroblast Serum Response Predicts Human Cancer Progression: Similarities between Tumors and Wounds. PLoS Biol 2004; 2(2):E7.
7. Tullai JW, Schaffer ME, Mullenbrock S et al. Immediate-early and delayed primary response genes are distinct in function and genomic architecture. J Biol Chem 2007; 282(33):23981-95
8. Li Z, Van Calcar S, Qu C et al. A global transcriptional regulatory role for c-Myc in Burkitt's lymphoma cells. Proc Natl Acad Sci USA 2003; 100(14):8164-8169.
9. Moreno-Bueno G, Cubillo E, Sarrio D et al. Genetic profiling of epithelial cells expressing e-cadherin repressors reveals a distinct role for snail, slug and e47 factors in epithelial-mesenchymal transition. Cancer Res 2006; 66(19):9543-9556.
10. Moreno-Bueno G, Sanchez-Estevez C, Cassia R et al. Differential gene expression profile in endometrioid and nonendometrioid endometrial carcinoma: STK15 is frequently overexpressed and amplified in nonendometrioid carcinomas. Cancer Res 2003; 63(18):5697-5702.
11. Winter SC, Buffa FM, Silva P et al. Relation of a hypoxia metagene derived from head and neck cancer to prognosis of multiple cancers. Cancer Res 2007; 67(7):3441-3449.
12. Nordsmark M, Bentzen SM, Rudat V et al. Prognostic value of tumor oxygenation in 397 head and neck tumors after primary radiation therapy. An international multi-center study. Radiother Oncol 2005; 77(1):18-24.
13. Zhao H, Kim Y, Wang P et al. Genome-wide characterization of gene expression variations and DNA copy number changes in prostate cancer cell lines. Prostate 2005; 63(2):187-197.
14. Bonaccorsi L, Muratori M, Carloni V et al. Androgen receptor and prostate cancer invasion. Int J Androl 2003; 26(1):21-25.
15. Sharpless NE, Chin L. The INK4a/ARF locus and melanoma. Oncogene 2003; 22(20):3092-3098.
16. Chin L, Merlino G, DePinho RA. Malignant melanoma: modern black plague and genetic black box. Genes Dev 1998; 12(22):3467-3481.
17. Cochran AJ. Prediction of outcome for patients with cutaneous melanoma. Pigment Cell Res 1997; 10(3):162-167.
18. Ahmed I. Malignant melanoma: prognostic indicators. Mayo Clin Proc 1997; 72(4):356-361.
19. Davies H, Bignell GR, Cox C et al. Mutations of the BRAF gene in human cancer. Nature 2002; 417(6892):949-954.
20. Omholt K, Karsberg S, Platz A et al. Screening of N-ras codon 61 mutations in paired primary and metastatic cutaneous melanomas: mutations occur early and persist throughout tumor progression. Clin Cancer Res 2002; 8(11):3468-3474.
21. Herlyn M, Satyamoorthy K. Activated ras. Yet another player in melanoma? Am J Pathol 1996; 149(3):739-744.
22. Schulze A, Nicke B, Warne PH et al. The transcriptional response to Raf activation is almost completely dependent on Mitogen-activated Protein Kinase Kinase activity and shows a major autocrine component. Mol Biol Cell 2004; 15(7):3450-3463.
23. Shields JM, Thomas NE, Cregger M et al. Lack of extracellular signal-regulated kinase mitogen-activated protein kinase signaling shows a new type of melanoma. Cancer Res 2007; 67(4):1502-1512.
24. Clark EA, Golub TR, Lander ES et al. Genomic analysis of metastasis reveals an essential role for RhoC. Nature 2000; 406(6795):532-535.

25. Wang W, Wyckoff JB, Goswami S et al. Coordinated regulation of pathways for enhanced cell motility and chemotaxis is conserved in rat and mouse mammary tumors. Cancer Res 2007; 67(8):3505-3511.
26. Bear JE, Roadcap DW. Unpublished Data. 2007.
27. Hasse A, Rosentreter A, Spoerl Z et al. Coronin 3 and its role in murine brain morphogenesis. Eur J Neurosci 2005; 21(5):1155-1168.
28. Berry M. Development of the cerebral neocortex of the rat. In: Gottlieb G, ed. Aspects of Neurogenesis. New York: Academic Press, 1974:Vol. 2. pp. 7-67.
29. Massey PV, Bashir ZI. Long-term depression: multiple forms and implications for brain function. Trends Neurosci 2007; 30(4):176-184.
30. Matsuzaki M, Honkura N, Ellis-Davies GC et al. Structural basis of long-term potentiation in single dendritic spines. Nature 2004; 429(6993):761-766.
31. Krucker T, Siggins GR, Halpain S. Dynamic actin filaments are required for stable long-term potentiation (LTP) in area CA1 of the hippocampus. Proc Natl Acad Sci USA 2000; 97(12):6856-6861.
32. Fukazawa Y, Saitoh Y, Ozawa F et al. Hippocampal LTP is accompanied by enhanced F-actin content within the dendritic spine that is essential for late LTP maintenance in vivo. Neuron 2003; 38(3):447-460.
33. Bjartmar C, Hildebrand C, Loinder K. Morphological heterogeneity of rat oligodendrocytes: Electron microscopic studies on serial sections. Glia 1994; 11:235-244.
34. Coffrey JC, McDermott KW. The regional distribution of myelin oligodendrocyte glycoprotein (MOG) in the developing rat CNS: An in vivo immunohistochemical study. J Neurocytol 1997; 26:149-161.
35. Weitzdoerfer R, Fountoulakis M, Lubec G. Reduction of actin-related protein complex 2/3 in fetal Down syndrome brain. Biochem Biophys Res Commun 2002; 293(2):836-841.
36. Neer EJ, Schmidt CJ, Smith T. LIS is more. Nat Genet 1993; 5(1):3-4.
37. Lo Nigro C, Chong CS, Smith AC et al. Point mutations and an intragenic deletion in LIS1, the lissencephaly causative gene in isolated lissencephaly sequence and Miller-Dieker syndrome. Hum Mol Genet 1997; 6(2):157-164.
38. Henning KA, Li L, Iyer N et al. The Cockayne syndrome group A gene encodes a WD repeat protein that interacts with CSB protein and a subunit of RNA polymerase II TFIIH. Cell 1995; 82(4):555-564.
39. Bassi MT, Ramesar RS, Caciotti B et al. X-linked late-onset sensorineural deafness caused by a deletion involving OA1 and a novel gene containing WD-40 repeats. Am J Hum Genet 1999; 64(6):1604-1616.
40. Tullio-Pelet A, Salomon R, Hadj-Rabia S et al. Mutant WD-repeat protein in triple-A syndrome. Nat Genet 2000; 26(3):332-335.
41. Handschug K, Sperling S, Yoon SJ et al. Triple A syndrome is caused by mutations in AAAS, a new WD-repeat protein gene. Hum Mol Genet 2001; 10(3):283-290.
42. Spoerl Z, Stumpf M, Noegel AA et al. Oligomerization, F-actin interaction and membrane association of the ubiquitous mammalian coronin 3 are mediated by its carboxyl terminus. J Biol Chem 2002; 277(50):48858-48867.
43. Thal DR, Xavier CP, Rosentreter A et al. Expression of coronin 3 in diffuse gliomas is related to malignancy. J Pathol. In press.
44. Kleihues P, Cavenee WK. Pathology and Genetics: Tumours of the Nervous System. Lyon: IARC-Press; 2000.
45. Foger N, Rangell L, Danilenko DM et al. Requirement for coronin 1 in T-lymphocyte trafficking and cellular homeostasis. Science 2006; 313(5788):839-842.
46. Yanagisawa Y, Sato Y, Asahi-Ozaki Y et al. Effusion and solid lymphomas have distinctive gene and protein expression profiles in an animal model of primary effusion lymphoma. J Pathol 2006; 209(4):464-473.
47. Graham SM, Vass JK, Holyoake TL et al. Transcriptional analysis of quiescent and proliferating CD34+ human haemopoietic cells from normal and CML sources. Stem Cells 2007; 25(12):3111-20.
48. Wilson CS, Davidson GS, Martin SB et al. Gene expression profiling of adult acute myeloid leukemia identifies novel biologic clusters for risk classification and outcome prediction. Blood 2006; 108(2):685-696.
49. Sasaki H, Nishikata I, Shiraga T et al. Overexpression of a cell adhesion molecule, TSLC1, as a possible molecular marker for acute-type adult T-cell leukemia. Blood 2005; 105(3):1204-1213.
50. Mahadevan D, Spier C, Della Croce K et al. Transcript profiling in peripheral T-cell lymphoma, not otherwise specified and diffuse large B-cell lymphoma identifies distinct tumor profile signatures. Mol Cancer Ther 2005; 4(12):1867-1879.
51. Ferrari G, Langen H, Naito M et al. A coat protein on phagosomes involved in the intracellular survival of mycobacteria. Cell 1999; 97(4):435-447.
52. Vergne I, Chua J, Singh SB et al. Cell biology of mycobacterium tuberculosis phagosome. Annu Rev Cell Dev Biol 2004; 20:367-394.

53. Anes E, Kuhnel MP, Bos E et al. Selected lipids activate phagosome actin assembly and maturation resulting in killing of pathogenic mycobacteria. Nat Cell Biol 2003; 5(9):793-802.
54. Deghmane AE, Soulhine H, Bach H et al. Lipoamide dehydrogenase mediates retention of coronin-1 on BCG vacuoles, leading to arrest in phagosome maturation. J Cell Sci 2007; 120(16):2796-806.
55. Jayachandran R, Sundaramurthy V, Combaluzier B et al. Survival of mycobacteria in macrophages is mediated by coronin 1-dependent activation of calcineurin. Cell 2007; 130(1):37-50.
56. Parekh AB, Putney JW Jr. Store-operated calcium channels. Physiol Rev 2005; 85(2):757-810.
57. Gallo EM, Cante-Barrett K, Crabtree GR. Lymphocyte calcium signaling from membrane to nucleus. Nat Immunol 2006; 7(1):25-32.
58. Cai L, Holoweckyj N, Schaller MD et al. Phosphorylation of coronin 1B by protein kinase C regulates interaction with Arp2/3 and cell motility. J Biol Chem 2005; 280(36):31913-31923.
59. Di Giovanni S, De Biase A, Yakovlev A et al. In vivo and in vitro characterization of novel neuronal plasticity factors identified following spinal cord injury. J Biol Chem 2005; 280(3):2084-2091.
60. Di Giovanni S, Knights CD, Rao M et al. The tumor suppressor protein p53 is required for neurite outgrowth and axon regeneration. EMBO J 2006; 25(17):4084-4096.
61. Martinez I, Lombardia L, Garcia-Barreno B et al. Distinct gene subsets are induced at different time points after human respiratory syncytial virus infection of A549 cells. J Gen Virol 2007; 88(Pt 2):570-581.
62. Fujimura N, Vacik T, Machon O et al. Wnt-mediated down-regulation of Sp1 target genes by a transcriptional repressor Sp5. J Biol Chem 2007; 282(2):1225-1237.
63. Hartman ZC, Kiang A, Everett RS et al. Adenovirus infection triggers a rapid, MyD88-regulated transcriptome response critical to acute-phase and adaptive immune responses in vivo. J Virol 2007; 81(4):1796-1812.
64. Pellagatti A, Cazzola M, Giagounidis AA et al. Gene expression profiles of CD34+ cells in myelodysplastic syndromes: involvement of interferon-stimulated genes and correlation to FAB subtype and karyotype. Blood 2006; 108(1):337-345.
65. Kakiuchi S, Daigo Y, Ishikawa N et al. Prediction of sensitivity of advanced nonsmall cell lung cancers to gefitinib (Iressa, ZD1839). Hum Mol Genet 2004; 13(24):3029-3043.
66. Hertel L, Mocarski ES. Global analysis of host cell gene expression late during cytomegalovirus infection reveals extensive dysregulation of cell cycle gene expression and induction of Pseudomitosis independent of US28 function. J Virol 2004; 78(21):11988-12011.
67. Ning W, Li CJ, Kaminski N et al. Comprehensive gene expression profiles reveal pathways related to the pathogenesis of chronic obstructive pulmonary disease. Proc Natl Acad Sci USA 2004; 101(41):14895-14900.
68. Chen H, Huang XN, Stewart AF et al. Gene expression changes associated with fibronectin-induced cardiac myocyte hypertrophy. Physiol Genomics 2004; 18(3):273-283.
69. Messmer D, Messmer B, Chiorazzi N. The global transcriptional maturation program and stimuli-specific gene expression profiles of human myeloid dendritic cells. Int Immunol 2003; 15(4):491-503.
70. Ross ME, Zhou X, Song G et al. Classification of pediatric acute lymphoblastic leukemia by gene expression profiling. Blood 2003; 102(8):2951-2959.

Index

A

Acanthamoeba 98-101
Actin 4, 6, 10, 11, 13, 15, 16, 21, 27, 31-38, 41, 49, 51, 52, 54, 56, 59, 61-67, 69, 72-85, 88-107, 110, 116, 120, 121, 124, 126, 129, 132
   Actin disassembly 61, 73, 76, 82, 83, 85
   Actin dynamics 33-35, 37, 38, 49, 72, 73, 75, 77, 83-85, 89, 98, 101, 102, 107, 116, 126, 129, 132
   Actin turnover 36, 38, 82, 83, 100, 129
Adaptor protein 14, 110, 113, 114
Ahcoronin 99
Aip1p 7, 10, 11, 15, 16
Arp2/3 4, 13, 14, 33-38, 56, 59, 62-65, 72-77, 79-81, 83-85, 100, 107, 116, 132
Arp2/3 Complex 4, 13, 14, 33-35, 38, 56, 62-65, 72-77, 79-81, 83-85, 100
ARPC1 7, 11, 13-15, 77
ATPs 36, 72, 76, 83, 84
Autoimmune disease 106
Axonal growth cone 93, 117

B

β-propeller 1, 2, 4, 6, 7, 9-11, 13-16, 20-24, 28, 32, 38, 41, 49, 56, 57, 59, 61, 62, 64-69, 73-75, 79-84, 88, 91, 92, 102, 105, 117, 118 s
β-TrCP 7, 13-15
Babesia 98, 100
Beta sheet 20-22
Biosynthetic pathway 110, 112, 113
Bootstrap confidence value 42
Brain development 5, 124, 126-128
Btb domains 14-16

C

Caenorhabditis elegan 4, 40, 57, 66, 71, 73, 86, 88, 90, 96-98, 110, 117
Calcineurin 37, 99, 106, 120, 121, 132
cAMP gradient 32, 91, 92
Cancer 4, 5, 27, 98, 102, 106, 124-126, 129, 130, 132

Cdc4p 7, 11, 13-15
Cdc42 98, 105, 106
Cell cycle 20, 21, 27
Cell motility 72, 75-77, 79-82, 85, 88, 89, 92, 102, 121, 124, 129
Chemotaxi 32, 37, 132
Cilia assembly 25
Clade 4, 41, 43, 45, 46
Cofilin 4, 32, 33, 35, 37, 62, 65, 66, 72, 73, 75, 76, 81-85, 100
Coiled coil domain 4, 41, 49, 56, 57, 59, 61-65, 95, 107, 116, 118-120
Comparative genomic 42, 52, 54
Computational biology 42
Coronin 5, 23, 27, 31-38, 41-47, 49-54, 56, 57, 59, 61-67, 69, 72-77, 79-85, 88-95, 98-107, 110-114, 116-121, 124-133
   Coronin 1 23, 47, 51, 56, 57, 59, 61-67, 69, 116-121, 129
   Coronin 1C 76, 77, 81, 124-128, 129-132
Coronin family 1, 15, 23, 31, 34, 36, 41, 51, 53, 73, 92, 94, 98
CRIB motif 105
Cullin ring ligase 14-16
Cytokinesis 32, 37, 53, 62, 72, 75, 76, 81, 85, 89, 91, 95, 100, 107
Cytoskeleton 4, 6, 16, 20, 21, 28, 32-35, 37, 38, 41, 46, 49, 62, 67, 72, 73, 76, 83, 88, 91-95, 101, 102, 105-107, 110, 120, 129

D

Dictyostelium discoideum 1, 31, 73, 88, 90, 102, 116
Dictyosteliums 1, 21, 25, 31, 32, 34, 37, 38, 43, 46, 51, 73, 76, 77, 88, 90, 91, 99-102, 105, 116, 117, 121
Domain organisation 66
Domains of unknown function (DUF) 41, 43, 54, 102
DUF1899 and DUF1900 41, 43, 44, 49, 51-53, 102

E

Electron microscopy 65, 79, 113, 117
Endocytosis 62, 72, 75, 76, 81, 85, 91, 93, 94, 107
Erk 125-127
Evolutionary conservation 42, 52, 53
Exon splicing 49

F

Fk506 120
Focal Adhesions 65, 103, 107
Folding Unit 61
Folds 4, 6, 7, 10, 11, 20-22, 28, 38, 59, 61, 64, 66, 76, 82, 83, 88, 117-119, 125
Functional Divergence 41

G

Galactose oxidase 10, 11
Gβ 7, 9, 11, 13, 32, 38
Green Fluorescent Protein (GFP) 33, 34, 37, 89, 91-99, 101
Glioma 5, 124, 129, 130
Golgi complex 4, 110, 112-114
Groucho/TLE 11, 13, 15

H

Hidden Markov Model (HMM) 23, 41, 42, 49-51, 102, 103
Homology model 2, 4, 62-64, 66, 105, 108
Human Gene Nomenclature Committee (HGNC) 45-47, 49, 99, 124

K

Katanin 15, 16
Keap1 7, 9-11, 13-16
Kelch 1, 6, 7, 9-11, 13-16, 107
KGD motif 49
Knockout 34, 35, 37, 102, 106
Kupffer cell 120

L

Lamellipodia 35, 62, 65, 76, 77, 85
Leucine zipper motif 101, 103
Leukocyte 4, 106, 116, 117, 120, 121
Lis1 7, 11, 13, 15, 16, 21, 25
Listeria 35, 82, 83, 106
Lymphocyte 21, 27, 75, 77, 80, 82, 132
Lysosome 37, 91, 106, 113, 120, 121, 130

M

Macrophage 34, 37, 79, 81, 91, 99, 101, 106, 117, 119-121, 130, 132
Maximum likelihood 42-44
Melanoma 5, 124-127, 129, 133
Metastasis 124-126
Microtubule 13, 15, 16, 25, 34, 36, 38, 46, 66, 73, 76, 85, 93, 100, 113
Mitochondrial 26, 37
Molecular docking 54
Molecular evolution 42
Multidomain 20, 22

N

Neutrophils 34, 35, 37, 77, 101, 106, 120
Nomenclature 1, 4, 41, 43, 45-47, 49, 50, 53, 56, 99, 102
Nrf2 13, 14

P

Pathogenic bacterial infection 124, 130, 132
PFAM database 103
Phagocytosis 21, 34, 36, 37, 75-77, 79, 89, 91, 92, 98-100, 102, 116, 120, 121, 130
Phagosome 34, 37, 91, 99, 101, 106, 120, 121, 130, 132
Phosphorylation 4, 35, 38, 56, 59, 62-66, 81, 85, 106, 107, 112, 114
Phylogenetic analysis 41, 43, 47, 49, 50, 52, 111
Plasmodium 98, 100, 101
Polarization 94, 95
Polymerization 31, 32, 34, 35, 77, 85, 88, 89
Protein interaction 5, 13, 14, 23, 26, 27, 38, 65, 73, 88, 107, 117

Protein transport 25, 114

R

Rac 98, 103, 105, 106
Ribosomal 21, 27
RNA processing 15, 20, 21, 28

S

Saccharomyces 73, 99, 103
Scruin 11, 15
Secondary structure prediction 4, 59, 62, 66
Sequence logo 49
Sequence threading 54
Signal transduction 16, 20, 21, 26-28, 92
Signature motif 57, 59, 61, 63, 64, 67
Single nucleotide polymorphism (SNP) 54
Slingshot phosphatase 35, 65
Species distribution 23, 41, 43, 45, 47, 49, 53, 54
Src 4, 66, 110, 112, 114
Stress fiber 85, 107
Structural domain 14, 49
Structural tetrad 59
Systemic lupus erythematosus (SLE) 106

T

3D modelling 1, 2, 4, 6, 7, 9-11, 13-16, 32, 38, 41, 49, 56, 57, 59, 61, 62, 64-69, 73-75, 79-84, 88, 91, 92, 102, 105, 117, 118
TACO 34, 47, 76, 120, 132
TFIID 21

Transcription 6, 14, 20, 21, 25, 28, 37, 106, 124, 125
Treadmilling 85
Trichomonas 46, 98, 100, 101, 103
Trimers 62, 63, 74, 117, 119

U

Ubiquitin 10, 11, 13, 14, 16, 20, 21, 26, 81

V

Vesicular trafficking 4, 20, 53, 98, 107
Villidin 4, 46, 51, 66, 89, 92, 100, 102, 103, 116
Virulence 98, 101, 102

W

Wd40 domain 41, 49, 51-53, 66, 93, 102, 117
Wd40 repeat 49, 56, 57
WD-repeat 22, 57
Whole genome duplication 41, 43, 52, 103, 104

X

Xenopus 42, 45, 76, 92, 98, 100-102, 104, 105

Z

Zebrafish 26, 42, 43, 92, 98, 103, 104